MAR 1 9 2024

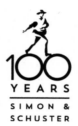
YEARS
SIMON & SCHUSTER

DEVOUT

A MEMOIR OF DOUBT

Anna Gazmarian

Simon & Schuster

NEW YORK   LONDON   TORONTO
SYDNEY   NEW DELHI

1230 Avenue of the Americas
New York, NY 10020

Some names and identifying characteristics have been changed.

This publication details the experiences of the author.
Readers should consult with their own medical or health
professionals about their own situations.

First Simon & Schuster hardcover edition March 2024

SIMON & SCHUSTER and colophon are registered trademarks
of Simon & Schuster, LLC

Simon & Schuster: Celebrating 100 Years of Publishing in 2024

For information about special discounts for bulk purchases,
please contact Simon & Schuster Special Sales at 1-866-506-1949
or business@simonandschuster.com.

The Simon & Schuster Speakers Bureau can bring authors to your
live event. For more information or to book an event, contact the
Simon & Schuster Speakers Bureau at 1-866-248-3049
or visit our website at www.simonspeakers.com.

Interior design by Paul Dippolito

Manufactured in the United States of America

1   3   5   7   9   10   8   6   4   2

Library of Congress Cataloging-in-Publication Data has been applied for.

ISBN 978-1-6680-0403-6
ISBN 978-1-6680-0405-0 (ebook)

For David and Ezra

Faith comes and goes. It rises and falls like the tides of an invisible ocean. If it is presumptuous to think that faith will stay with you forever, it is just as presumptuous to think that unbelief will.

—*Flannery O'Connor*

Note: This memoir is a work of creative nonfiction. I have reconstructed my memories and conversations to the best of my ability. For the sake of the story, some characters have been combined and renamed. My intention is to show the complicated intersection between religion and mental illness. I wish to capture every person truthfully.

Preface

At three months old I was baptized in Mount Airy, North Carolina, a town where my dad is a local celebrity for his love of exercise, running up to six miles on the side of the road during his lunch breaks, and where *The Andy Griffith Show* was filmed. Here, walking down the street often means running into your next-door neighbors and dentist. This is one of the reasons why my introverted parents from Michigan ended up resettling into the larger suburb of Winston-Salem from Mount Airy: they wanted more privacy. They also wanted more school options. In the photo of my baptism, my mother, trying to keep my lace-patterned silk dress from getting wet, holds me while a pastor sprinkles water over my head. In the Christian faith, a baptism symbolizes a believer's faith in Jesus, the ultimate sign of death to sin, the burial of an old life. Jesus says in scripture to have the faith and wonder of a child. Maybe this is what he means.

My evangelical Christian community was the center of my upbringing, the organizing principle around which everything else in my life was ordered. Even as a kid, though, I struggled with whether my faith was all it could and should be. After all, I'd been baptized without my conscious consent. Another way of saying this is that my faith lacked agency.

I was determined to be a good Christian, but I struggled with doubt. In my community, doubt wasn't welcome. I learned this the hard way, as an eight-year-old watching a live-action Christian TV show called *Bibleman*, in which Doubt is a personified villain with a cape, the archnemesis of the show's hero, who has a six-pack. Bibleman himself was modeled after Batman, except that he was a devout Christian who fought doubt and sin. The message was clear: Doubt was an enemy.

As a freshman in college, I decided to be rebaptized by my high school youth pastor, a man named Jason who helped lead a church that met weekly in a middle school auditorium. I believed that my baptism as an adult would relieve me of doubts and clarify my purpose in life. Six months after my baptism, I was diagnosed with bipolar disorder.

My life has never been the same. But almost as painful as the loss of my mental health was the loss of a coherent worldview that was rooted in my faith. From that day on, I've been breaking down and rebuilding my concept of faith, searching for a faith that can exist alongside doubt, a faith that is built on trust rather than fear. A faith with room for prayer and lament. That's what this book is: a prayer and a lament, offered in the hope of restoration.

Chapter 1

During my first psychiatric evaluation in November 2011, my psychiatrist, Dr. Ferguson, picked up a dark wooden pen from her glass desk and cleared her throat.

"Can you describe what brought you here today?"

Before this appointment, I visited the library at Wake Forest University to read through a copy of the *DSM*, commonly used by psychiatrists to diagnose people with mental illnesses. As I watched students studying at long table tables, I read about how depression is scientifically defined. I was seeking a definition separate from what my church taught about depression, which had to do with spiritual fitness and possible demonic activity. I expected my appointment to involve a quick diagnosis of major depressive disorder before sending me out the door with a stack of prescriptions from a doctor I'd never see again.

I told Dr. Ferguson about how I'd lost my job at a coffee shop in my hometown of Winston-Salem, North Carolina; about how I'd slept through freshman finals and never wrote assigned research papers; about how I'd taken a leave of absence for my sophomore fall semester; and about how, without trying, in the four months leading up to this visit, I'd lost twenty pounds.

"Have you tried any other treatments?" she asked.

I took out a wrinkled piece of paper on which I'd written down the name of the drug my primary care doctor had prescribed five months earlier: CYMBALTA. Classified as an SSRI (selective serotonin reuptake inhibitor), Cymbalta is a drug whose purpose is to boost serotonin and norepinephrine in the brain. When serotonin and norepinephrine are at normal levels, they help with emotional stability and allow the body to manage stress reactions. It's not surprising that a doctor would think I needed this kind of help. But Cymbalta comes with many side effects, too, and in the five months since I'd started taking it, I'd experienced every single one: nausea, drowsiness, headaches, brain fog, loss of appetite, excessive sweating, and fatigue. It can also increase suicidal thinking, especially among people under twenty-four—put a check next to that, too. Whenever I drove my car, I'd taken to imagining driving straight off the road; I was frequently pulling into random parking lots just to breathe. All this is what led me to schedule an initial psychiatry appointment.

Something else brought me to Dr. Ferguson, too—the fact that my months of work with my Christian therapist, Claudia, had failed to lift me out of this state. Claudia engaged in what's known as "biblical counseling," a branch of Christian therapy in which a clinician uses the Bible to interpret your mental and emotional health. In biblical counseling, the basics of psychology are discarded, dismissed as secular. This made sense enough to me; like many other Christians I knew, I had a learned skepticism about anything overly "scientific."

Claudia's chin-length hair was as white as the pearl necklace she always wore, and she smelled like a mix of potpourri and the six cats she owned. Every Wednesday at ten a.m., I sat in the basement of her two-story house, located twenty minutes from where I lived, and sought spiritual comfort. She opened each session with a prayer for me to feel peace. My goal for those sessions was to find some relief, any relief, from what felt like unending suffering. Claudia pointed me to scripture verses and taught me prayers that she thought might help me. If only I said the right words, or read the right things, or thought the right thoughts, then maybe God would help me. In all the time that I saw her, Claudia never mentioned the possibility of mental illness.

During one session, Claudia noticed that I appeared distressed, and she picked up the Bible and started reading to me from the Book of Psalms. The Book of Psalms is an anthology of songs that have been recited and sung by people and communities throughout history, and it's broken into five major types: thanksgiving psalms, royalty psalms, wisdom psalms, lament psalms, and praise psalms. Claudia read from one of the thanksgiving psalms. " 'So rejoice in the Lord and be glad, you righteous,' " she read. " 'Sing, all you who are upright in heart!' " I was familiar with this type of message; psalms of thanksgiving were the most common type I heard every Sunday morning during my worship services. But despite this familiarity, this sentiment felt inaccessible to me when I was depressed.

Claudia looked at me to see if I appeared encouraged. My

shoulders caved in as I leaned forward on the velvet couch— definitely not encouraged. It occurred to me the verse she read would make sense on a Christian greeting card. When I realized she was waiting to see a reaction, I clasped my hands, trying to appear at ease. I didn't know how to ask Claudia how I could rejoice in the Lord and be glad, or be upright in heart, if my life seemed meaningless. Neither Claudia nor anyone else in my religious community ever discussed this with me.

For years I kept prayer journals and made lists of all the sins I believed I'd committed. Working with Claudia, I kept doing this, only more so. I became obsessive. I wrote down, in excruciating detail, every thought pertaining to the ways I hoped to die. Everywhere I went involved noticing various methods I could use to take my own life. But because I feared what conclusions she might reach about me if I mentioned my suicidal thoughts, I never shared them with her; I sat across from her each week and did as I was told.

After two months of working with Claudia, I spent a weekend at Well of Mercy, a religious center owned by a group of nuns. People paid whatever they could afford to go there, and received the added bonus of home-cooked meals. I used the last one hundred dollars from my paycheck from the coffee shop to stay there for two nights. I had intended to use that time to pray and read, but instead I spent most of my time sleeping in a hammock. As a last-ditch effort to cleanse myself once and for all, I wrote out my sins on porcelain plates and smashed them in a graveyard, a suggestion I read in a Christian blog. Smashing plates is also a tradition at weddings, symbolizing a new beginning. But I was not cleansed. Spiritual retreats and rituals were proving insufficient. I needed medical support. I called Dr. Ferguson.

As I took off my shoes and curled into a ball on her leather couch, Dr. Ferguson stared at her computer screen and typed, taking breaks only to jot notes in a manila folder marked with my name.

"Have you had any suicidal thoughts?" she asked.

At that point in my life, my understanding was that God sent people who committed suicide to hell. I was concerned that my suicidal ideations—thoughts of driving off the road or taking an entire bottle of pills—ensured my damnation. So, I lied to Dr. Ferguson the same way I'd lied to Claudia.

Twirling a few strands of her long gray hair with her finger, Dr. Ferguson got up from her desk and looked through a filing cabinet. "Aha!" she said. She grabbed a blue folder with a white label with something illegible scrawled on it. She took a handout from the folder before placing it on my lap. I'll never know how she reached the conclusion that this sheet was what I needed to read. It read "What Is Type Two Bipolar?" She had arrived at a diagnosis.

Bipolar II is marked by a cycle of hypomanic and depressive symptoms, and is slightly less severe than bipolar I. The sheet I held in my hand informed me that "hypomanic" is a milder form of mania that typically lasts for shorter amounts of time compared to full-blown mania—but can still seem quite manic. Mania, I learned, was marked by signs of erratic behavior and days without sleep. Dr. Ferguson explained that mania sometimes includes periods of complete obsession with and absorption by certain activities.

Several of my experiences started to come into focus: staying up all night to paint in my mom's studio, spontaneously driving to the beach in the middle of the night. Had I done these things because of an undiagnosed mental illness? Or were they just part of my personality? I was known among my friends for my passion and enthusiasm. Were these, too, a result of bipolar? I couldn't parse this out.

"Can this disease just appear out of thin air?" I asked.

Dr. Ferguson went on to explain a concept in psychiatry known as the "diathesis-stress model," which suggests that mental illness can emerge in people with certain genetic predispositions when exposed to all-consuming stressors. She explained that it was possible that my on-again, off-again relationship with a psychology major, my mom's health scares, and my obsession with acing each of my classes led to a perfect storm for a mental health crisis. I also knew from my psychology classes that there is sometimes a hereditary component to mental illness; I didn't know if my grandfather had ever received a diagnosis, but I did know he had died by suicide. Left unaddressed at that point, but what has become clearer to me in time, is that my religious ideas had played a role in this crisis, too.

"I noticed on your paperwork," Dr. Ferguson said, "that you were diagnosed with ADHD in elementary school. It's not uncommon for people to have ADHD as well as bipolar. Their symptoms overlap."

Research since then has borne this out. A 2021 study in *Medicina* found that comorbidity for adults with bipolar and ADHD is as high as 20 percent. A meta-analysis of several studies published in *Neuroscience & Biobehavioral Review* found that one in thirteen adults with ADHD is also diagnosed with bipolar disorder. Both conditions share symptoms like impulsivity, distractibility, lack of focus, and an inability to relax.

I'd received my ADHD diagnosis in fourth grade after teachers expressed concerns about the fact that I could never sit still in class and that I could never seem to stop talking. I'd been on medication ever since, cycling on and off different drug combinations all the way through high school. I hated the thought of having to repeat this process in college. Sitting there in Dr. Ferguson's office, my mind grappled with two painful, unanswerable questions. How would my body handle another diagnosis and more medication? And why did God allow me to have abnormal brain chemistry?

My religious community believed in spiritual warfare, the idea that demonic and angelic forces were constantly at work in this life. Whenever anyone in my church died by suicide, struggled with addiction, or got pregnant before marriage, Satan was responsible. God and Satan were talked about as if they were a long-standing sports rivalry. When responding to questions about why suffering existed, church leaders in my community tended to blame the pain in our lives on Satan or sin rather than admit that there were things that happened in this world that we had no logical explanation for.

Throughout the Bible, several individuals are filled with demons who, like Satan, were fallen angels who have rebelled against God, resulting in their being sent to hell. There's one story in particular that proved especially challenging to me after my diagnosis. It is recounted in three books in the New Testament: Matthew, Mark, and Luke, referred to as the synoptic Gospels, or the Gospels that tell the same general story of the life of Jesus. I have studied scripture since preschool, when parents taught weekly lessons and sang songs based around the Bible. These stories have shaped my worldview and how I live my life. I speak of the characters in present tense, as if they are close friends, because of how intertwined their lives feel with mine. In this particular story, Jesus walks along the Sea of Galilee, preaching, healing, and performing miracles with his disciples. At one point he encounters a man in apparent distress, a man who lives "among the tombs." Each Gospel writer makes clear that this man's anguish is caused by demonic possession. When the man sets his eyes on Jesus, he runs toward him and bows before him, begging not to be tormented further. Jesus looks upon the man with mercy and commands the demons to leave him at once. The demons obey, and upon fleeing the man, they enter a herd of nearby pigs. The pigs then rush down a bank and drown themselves in the sea.

The man, in other words, is healed. People from throughout the area flock to him, eager to witness this miracle of healing. How did this man, once so frightening, become restored to sanity? As Jesus prepares to leave, the man asks for permission to follow him. But Jesus tells him instead to stay and reveal to his friends what the Lord has done for him.

Reading this story after my diagnosis, I tried to make logical sense of it, to put a diagnosis on the man. Was the demon a mental illness that, because of the religious rituals of the time, went undiagnosed? Were demons the designated language? What always confused me is how the demon got there to begin with and why God allowed the man to be possessed. I believed that a dark spirit world existed within our realm of existence. To avoid these forces of evil, I stayed clear of tarot cards, Harry Potter, and psychic readings. I feared being possessed by a demon and prayed every night, even in college, for God to protect me against the forces of evil. But around the time of my diagnosis, I experienced vivid nightmares of my body falling through an abyss and landing in a pit of molten lava. *Is it God communicating through my dreams, or is it Satan?* The uncertainty scared me.

The most cited example about evil playing a role in suffering comes from the story of Job. In the book of Job, Satan appears before God after looking upon the earth. The Lord asks Satan if he noticed Job, a man with complete integrity and blamelessness. Satan questions whether Job's faithfulness to God is tied to the blessings in his life. He tells God that if everything is taken away, Job will turn his back on his faith.

God agrees to test Job as Satan suggests, because he knows that nothing Satan can do will cause Job to lose faith. First, God allows Satan to cause Job to lose his property and children. Job responds by tearing off his clothes to express his agony and yet still blesses the Lord. Satan inflicts Job with sores all over his body. In his physical suffering, Job curses the day of his birth and yet he continues to pray while seeking out God's wisdom for his life beyond his own understanding. Scripture does not address how long Job suffered, if his anguish lasted days, weeks, months, or years. Despite Job's agony and endless questions, God still deems him faithful, because he continues to wrestle with his faith through prayer despite his painful circumstances. Eventually, God restores what Job lost. With the story of Job in the back of my mind, I wondered if my bipolar disorder diagnosis was a test of my faith and held out hope that if I, like Job, refused to curse my maker, my diagnosis would disappear, and I would no longer have thoughts of killing myself.

Before I asked any other questions, Dr. Ferguson stressed that bipolar disorder had a high suicide rate, one of the highest of all mental illnesses. She told me about a popular study published by *Bipolar Disorders* in 2010 that estimated that between 20 and 60 percent of individuals with bipolar attempted suicide at least once in their lifetime. The likelihood was increased for those who did not take medications. "It's so important for you to take your medications as prescribed. Will you promise me not to miss any dosages?" she said. I vowed never to miss a dosage, fearing that doing so would cause my thoughts of death to become even more overwhelming. She continued telling me about mortality rates for people with bipolar disorder. Dr. Ferguson said that a 2011 study published in *Schizophrenia Research* discovered that life expectancy for women with bipolar disorder was more than twelve years shorter than that of the average person. But Dr. Ferguson assured me that taking medication could help improve that number.

Though I couldn't go a day without thinking about my own death, I didn't want to die, and I promised Dr. Ferguson that I would keep attending appointments for the sake of my own life. Dr. Ferguson pulled out her wooden pen, wrote the prescriptions for two mood stabilizers—Lamictal and Cymbalta, despite experiencing an array of side effects—and told me to return in two weeks.

Chapter 2

Arriving back from my appointment, I walked across the concrete driveway belonging to the white stucco house that I had
called my home since kindergarten. After placing my keys on
the granite kitchen counter, I ran downstairs to find my mom
painting in her art studio.

"I think that I figured out what's wrong with me," I said,
handing her the bipolar pamphlets. She dropped the paint-
brush that she was holding and scanned the document.

"Does having a diagnosis," my mom wondered aloud,
"give you comfort to explain what's been going on with you?"

Before looking up from her painting, she removed streaks
of paint from her highlighted hair. The flecks of turquoise and
red belonged to a landscape that she was working on. When her
green eyes met mine, they appeared brighter than the fluorescents
in her studio. Until I handed her the pamphlets, my mother iden-
tified ways in which I wasn't like myself. I usually had a sense of
humor and a social life spent hanging out with friends at coffee
shops or exploring downtown, but by that point, I spent most
days in bed, leaving texts and phone calls unanswered. Normally,
I came downstairs in the evenings to watch *Grey's Anatomy* and
home decorating shows with her and my father, but recently I
chose instead to remain in the confines of my room.

Because she was the type of person who found a positive spin to almost everything, when I shared my fear regarding my diagnosis, her only response, made while rubbing her hands against gray sweatpants covered in years-old paint, was *God will never put you through something that you can't handle.* Her offered encouragement came from a popular mantra in our Christian community. They put a positive spin on hardships as a form of spiritual growth. But my brain worked much differently than my mother's or anyone else in my church. Instead of being encouraged, I thought of how I had recently attended the funeral of a friend whose dad died by suicide. During the service, I held her on the bathroom floor as she cried. Did God give him more than what he could handle? Did he just not have enough faith, or was it more complicated than that? I did not know the answer.

What my mom shared with me is part of a pattern that she learned from her identification as an evangelical, which in Greek literally translates to "good news." That meant that no matter what I shared, my mother, being a woman of good news, would always find a bright spot. I left the basement without offering another word.

* * *

The ability to find hope and happiness in whatever life throws at Christians in my community is central to how faith was taught to me as a child. In Sunday school, we studied the fruits of the spirit, nine attributes that many Christians in my community saw as a sign of God at work in their lives. In the book of Galatians, a letter addressed to Christians in Galatia,

Apostle Paul lists the fruits of the spirit as love, joy, peace, forbearance, kindness, goodness, faithfulness, gentleness, and self-control. Paul describes these attributes as gifts from the Holy Spirit to followers of Christ. When I was a child, they felt like items to check from a list to determine if my life adhered to an authentic Christian moral framework. If a professed Christian around me did not outwardly exhibit fruitfulness in his or her life, such as kindness or self-control, others in my community called these fruitless people's faith into question.

Teachers wrote the words on cutout drawings of fruit for our classroom, a simple craft paper map for how I was to achieve God's love and approval and earn eternal life. I obsessively ate grapes, strawberries, and mangoes in hopes of becoming more patient and joyful as a child in Sunday school even though the spiritual fruits Paul spoke of weren't actual, literal food. Positive emotions seemed like signals that I was following the plan that God had laid out for my life. But I worried in my depression that my inability to see my diagnosis as good news, that the lack of fruit in my life, meant that I was going to hell, that I was an unbeliever of God, just like the rest of the world. My ruminating over death did not push me closer to experiencing fruits like peace or forbearance. Instead, I felt turmoil. Caught up in tracing my shortcomings, I did not recognize the faith that I was displaying in getting myself the treatment that I needed.

A week after my mother's misguided attempt at comforting me with her good news, I visited Seth, my high school youth pastor, at his house in the hopes of finding encouragement about my diagnosis. I anticipated that his words might lead me to the peace and joy that I often saw in my parents. Given his track record of preferring to play games over having deep discussions about life, I was nervous about the conversation.

I would have gone to my college pastor, Jason, but he wasn't an option. The recent fallout with my ex-boyfriend, who had been offered an internship with him, resulted in my college pastor asking me to step down from the leadership team and leave the church. Jason worried that my depression and lingering feelings for my ex distracted him from strengthening his relationship with God.

I texted Seth ahead of time about my diagnosis, and he was quick to respond that I was in his family's thoughts and prayers. Arriving at his house, I found him sweeping off his front porch in one of the V-neck shirts our youth group sold to raise money for our annual summer mission trip to Estonia. As I parked in the driveway, I saw him wipe sweat from his brow and wave. Seth opened the front door and led me through several rooms in his house to show me different projects he worked on, like regrouting the tile backsplash in his kitchen. I noticed as he spoke that, since I had arrived, he had not looked at me once.

Finally, he led me to his back porch and shared stories about his mentally ill mother-in-law. Her exact diagnosis and circumstances went over my head, but I remember him leaning his head back and laughing, voicing annoyance over her constant anxiety and depression about her situation.

"She's crazy!" Then he looked straight at me. "She never knows how to look at the bright side of things like Christians do."

My stomach turned to knots because I knew exactly what he meant and worried that he thought the same of me. What he suggested connected with how my mom had initially approached my diagnosis. Suffering Christians in my community were supposed to handle their circumstances with a level of positivity that I lacked. To me, it sounded as though he believed that his mother-in-law's mental health state could be attributed to her inability to put a positive spin on her lifelong health problems.

Throughout my involvement in church, pastors served as middlemen between God and their congregants. I believed their position of power gave them authority over me, and I respected and trusted each of them. But when Seth referred to his mother-in-law as "crazy," I realized that, after knowing him for five years and looking to him for spiritual direction, I could no longer trust him. This confirmed my suspicions from years prior, back when, as a high schooler, I'd sought his counsel. When I told him about my anxiety, he reminded me, "We are called to cast our anxieties onto Jesus. Give all your worries to him!"

A few days after my trip to Seth's house, I arrived at church, wondering what those around me would say if they learned of my diagnosis. Thanks to the weight loss and the impulsive decision to cut off my hair with craft scissors, my friends already believed me unhealthy. Despite having slept only three hours, I piled on concealer underneath my eyes to appear alert and awake. When my mom saw that I wasn't singing along with the worship music like I normally did, she put her arm around me.

My parents prioritized raising my sister and me within a Christian community because they wanted to teach us faith values in ways that differed from their own upbringings, where religion was treated more casually. Neither of my parents grew up evangelical, and they both describe their early church experiences as being more of a social gathering. As newlyweds, they attended church together and viewed it more as a part of their weekly routine rather than a matter of deep conviction.

By the time I turned ten, we switched over to attending a nondenominational church when my older sister, Allie, was in middle school so that she could have a youth group. On Sunday mornings, when I wanted to sleep in, my parents reminded me that church was not optional in our household.

Nondenominational churches like the one we attended have the freedom not to follow strict theological doctrines. This is partly why they tend to attract people with religious baggage: the congregations appear to offer complete abandonment from the confines of a particular denomination and to focus solely on the pure teachings of Christ. My mom remained active as a youth group leader, my father led small groups, and we traveled on international mission trips together. The churches we attended always served as our home and community. We met throughout my life on Sunday mornings in high school gymnasiums, middle school auditoriums, and new buildings that cost large amounts that I could not fathom. Hundreds of families around town attended these services each week.

* * *

During the first church service right after my diagnosis, a pastor, Michael, took the stage to give his testimony. This was the leader's first time back among the congregation after he'd checked into a Christian rehabilitation center for alcoholism and drug addiction. Our congregation had paid for his stay. He wore the unofficial uniform of pastors in our congregation: black Chuck Taylors, an oversize flannel shirt, and tight jeans. His hair stood up like porcupine quills from the amount of wax he used. Michael put his hands in his dark jean pockets and said, "I was diagnosed with bipolar disorder during my rehabilitation."

This revelation piqued my interest, causing me to sit up in my chair. For the first time since talking to Dr. Ferguson, I felt a moment of hope and connection. But as Michael paced the stage and looked out into the crowd, his testimony took an expected turn.

"My sin has hurt my family, and I'm sorry."

As Michael took his hands and wiped away the tears from his eyes, his gold wedding ring glistened. His wife, wearing a jean jacket over a long dress, took the stage for a moment to give him a hug. She wrapped her arms around him as he buried his head against her shoulder, and they both tried to hold back tears. Looking over at my parents, I felt a small pang of guilt, wondering how much pain my depression caused them. My pastor's narrative made it seem like his struggles, rather than being caused by a clinical disease or a biological predisposition, were the fault of his decisions alone. While there was a part of me that thought about pulling my pastor aside to tell him his diagnosis wasn't his fault and his message was one I needed to hear myself, I walked straight to the car after the service without acknowledging anyone.

* * *

Later in the story of Job, after he's lost everything in his life, he goes to his three friends, Eliphaz, Bildad, and Zophar, for comfort. They sit with him for seven days and seven nights without saying a word to him, being present as Job grieves his losses and processes his suffering. To show solidarity, they weep with him, tearing their robes and throwing dust in the air and letting it settle upon their heads.

But after seven days, they become impatient with him. They want him to move on with his life. Each friend begins offering him advice. Eliphaz, the first to speak, suggests that Job suffered because he sinned against God. He believes that if Job committed more of his life to God, then his suffering would cease. Bildad speaks next, explaining that Job lost his children because they were punished for their own sins. Zophar questions if Job was as blameless as he appeared, since it seems clear that Job is being punished for something. Each of these friends' responses to Job's suffering represents common explanations in the Christian communities where I grew up for why suffering exists—placing personal responsibility and guilt on those who suffer.

I connected to Job feeling the weight of everyone offering advice and counsel for why everything was going wrong in his life. The same seemed to be happening in mine. Many of my closest friends who knew that I had been struggling for months told me to be joyful, to pray more often, to look at the bright side, to count my blessings. My depression was increasingly being treated as the result of not being able to feel gratitude in my life.

When God finally addresses Job's questions, he offers a long-winded speech about the mysteries and wonders of the universe. God asks Job impossible questions, like *Were you there when I laid the earth's foundations?* The point is clear enough: Job is not God. Job is fallible. Job is not the center of the universe. There's a lot that happens—even in Job's life—that has nothing to do with Job.

God puts Job's suffering in a larger context, revealing how God is intimately involved in every detail of our world, including our individual lives. God reminds Job about how he was present over the creation of the earth, the foundation being poured, and the stars being set in the sky. God answers Job's pleas indirectly by showing how he is active in the universe, even in Job's life, even in Job's pain. Job responds not with more questions but by acknowledging his own insignificance in the universe. Despite Job's questions and anguish, God views Job as faithful and restores his losses. What takes me aback is that God never answers Job's questions directly about why his suffering existed, and yet he still chooses to praise him. Throughout his suffering, Job does not allow the silence he felt from God to fill him with bitterness that kept him from seeking after him. He never stops crying out to God for help. I prayed that I could do the same in my own journey—like Job, with more questions than answers.

* * *

My pastor's testimony reinforced the idea in my mind that depression could be alleviated by a simple change of mindset. What I struggled with daily was seen by many in my community as the result of choosing to look at the world through a negative lens. A text from a good friend read: "Just try to be happy!"

It's difficult to define how my community approached mental illness when the term is used interchangeably in sermons and worship songs with words like *hopelessness*, *despair*, and *sorrow*. Regardless, many of those closest to me treated depression as a spiritual ailment. When I heard a friend give her faith testimony, she compared having depression with demonic possession. She claimed that her prayer life and church community saved her from emotional pain, enabling her to go off psychiatric medications.

A week after my pastor's testimony, I was scheduled to attend a holiday party with a group of friends from my high school. We attended a Southern Baptist high school together and bonded over surviving the numerous rules and scandals, like the time swimmers got high on cough syrup or the time our principal got fired for drinking wine with his wife at an Italian restaurant.

The plan was for me to drive to my friend Sarah's house, do our makeup, and get dressed before heading over to the party. On my drive there, my phone died, and I realized that I had no idea where I was going. Finally, I recognized a playground nearby my friend's house and showed up nearly two hours late.

She opened her door and ran out, looking terrified. "Are you okay? I was worried that something had happened." Though I wanted to tell her about my diagnosis, my shame prevented me from doing so.

The same day I told my mom about my diagnosis, days before getting lost on my way to Sarah's house, I delivered the news to my dad over dinner as soon as he got home from his management job at a steel company. Placing his hands on my shoulders, he brought me in close and told me that he and my mom would pay for whatever treatment I needed.

"We should get a second opinion."

Chapter 3

Moments before my two-week follow-up appointment with Dr. Ferguson, I sat on a wooden bench across from her office, filling out a mood chart. A mood chart is what behavioral health providers often ask patients to use in order to track different emotions, symptoms, and external factors to get a better gauge of where to go with treatment. The sheet asked me to rate each symptom on a scale from zero to four. Since my initial appointment, she insisted on having me fill these out before we met because she wanted to see if the medications were working or if adjustments needed to be made. Questions on the chart focused on issues like my ability to have interest in things I normally enjoyed, excessive worrying, difficulty falling asleep, inability to concentrate, agitation, and anxiety. Zero on the scale meant not at all, and four indicated extremely common.

Rubbing lotion into her hands, Dr. Ferguson walked out of her office, asking if I was ready. I handed her my sheet, where I had circled four for every answer. As she reviewed my answers from her desk, she grabbed a celery stick from a reusable blue container. Dr. Ferguson placed the vegetable in her mouth like a cigar, the crunch of her celery and the ticking from the grandfather clock the only sounds in the otherwise silent room.

"Why didn't you fill anything in at, like, a two?"

"Because I only feel emotions at either a zero or a four; there's no middle ground."

"Based on how you've been rating your depression, we're going to have to increase your Lamictal and add another medication."

Prior to that appointment, I took Cymbalta and Lamictal each morning to manage my mood, never missing a dosage. Per her suggestions, I also took fish oil, yellow capsules that caused me to have burps that tasted like salmon. According to a 2011 meta-analysis in *The Journal of Clinical Psychiatry*, omega-3 can improve bipolar symptoms for individuals because of how fish oil can activate anti-inflammatory mechanisms in the brain. I did not notice a difference but continued to take the oversize capsules that stuck to the back of my throat each day no matter how much water I drank. Lamictal is a medication designed originally for those with epilepsy to help treat epileptic seizures but is also used for those with bipolar disorder in helping delay mood episodes. The drug is one that doctors must gradually increase because of the side effects. It comes with risks of a life-threatening skin rash, slurred speech, confusion, increased sensitivity to light, and acne. She pulled out her computer and scheduled me for another two-week follow-up.

* * *

In the weeks between our second and third visits, I read stories of Christ's miracles. One of my favorite miracles takes place in each of the synoptic Gospels. Each account tells the story of a woman who bled for twelve years. Her name is not mentioned in scripture. Many scholars interpret her health condition to be menorrhagia, menstrual bleeding that lasts longer than seven days. The book of Leviticus establishes that women on their periods during biblical times were considered unclean and, therefore, anyone who touched them was also considered unclean. A woman who bled for as long as this woman bled would've been deemed a social outcast.

One day, as she sees Jesus walking through town, she runs toward him, making her way through a crowd of followers and onlookers, and touches the hem of his garment. Scripture provides no account of her inner logic; we're left to wonder why she chose to do this. Perhaps she had heard about Jesus performing other miracles throughout Jerusalem and thought that touching him would be enough to heal her. She had suffered for so long; she surely must have felt desperate.

At the time, Jesus is on his way with his disciples to see Jarius, a synagogue leader whose daughter has died. When the woman touches his cloak, he feels power go out of him. "Who touched me?" he asks. The woman steps forward and falls at his feet, admitting to what had happened: an act of complete desperation. Jesus tells her, "Daughter, your faith has healed you. Go in peace and be freed from your suffering" (Mark 5:34). The Gospels tell us that she was healed from that day on.

I related to this woman's desperation and her desire for wholeness. Through medication, I wondered, could Dr. Ferguson do for me what Jesus did for this woman? Was healing possible? Dr. Ferguson told me that I would always experience bipolar symptoms and that the medications were necessary to help me live a functional life. Bipolar disorder is not an illness that disappears with proper treatment. But at the time of my diagnosis, I had not accepted the lifelong prognosis and wanted a miracle from God—God, and Dr. Ferguson. I prayed each night for a miracle of biblical proportions that exceeded the logic of scientific study, for my medical case to be unlike anything that my doctor had seen before. I fell asleep each night praying that one day I would no longer have to reach for the orange pill bottles each morning.

* * *

I learned at a young age that I could make my life better by turning to God in prayer, Bible reading, and loving other people. But now I was turning to Dr. Ferguson to fix me. She had faith, too—faith in medications to work a particular way.

In general, mood stabilizers are designed to help prevent further manic episodes and keep depression from becoming debilitating. No cure for mental illness exists. Instead, working with doctors is a matter of finding the best combination possible that makes living life more bearable. According to a 1995 study published in *The American Journal of Psychiatry*, even with treatment, 37 percent of individuals with bipolar disorder relapse by experiencing depressive or manic episodes within one year, 60 percent within two years. In an article in the *Archives of General Psychiatry* published in 2002, scientists found that after the initial onset, patients with bipolar experience depressive symptoms for about a third of the weeks of their life, although this differs from person to person. Even with the uncertainty of medications, the alternatives are even more risky. While drugs can delay manic and depressive episodes, not having stabilizers can result in more frequent mania and depression. These episodes can decrease brain size and certain areas of the brain. Gray matter in the brain is destroyed with every manic or depressive episode. This part of the brain is important for memory and emotional regulation. A history of bipolar disorder increases the risk of dementia, but medications have the ability to lessen this risk.

After Dr. Ferguson increased my Lamictal in my second appointment, I noticed that my speech became slurred. During normal conversations with friends and family, I began mixing words together. My tongue felt stuck to the top of my mouth. Whenever this happened, my friends either laughed or asked me to repeat myself. I began rehearsing everything that I said before speaking, hoping to prevent my words from flowing together.

In our next appointment together, I paced around Dr. Ferguson's office and told her about the latest side effect. She encouraged me to wait it out to see if improvements happened. I held the back of the chair where I normally sat and looked at her.

"Can you give me a timeline for when I will feel better?"

"Finding the correct drug cocktail is trial and error. Some of these drugs take months to reach their full effect. None of this is predictable."

For the next two weeks, I was to take the same dosage of Lamictal, despite the side effects, along with Doxepin once a day. Dr. Ferguson said it would take two to three weeks for me to notice a difference in my medication changes. She noticed my sunken shoulders when she revealed this timeline and told me to be patient. She crossed her legs before revealing that Doxepin comes with a warning that during clinical studies, young adults became suicidal. It is classified as a tricyclic antidepressant that focuses on norepinephrine. These drugs have been used less often by psychiatrists since the introduction of SSRIs and SNRIs (serotonin-norepinephrine reuptake inhibitors) in the 1980s. Already debating whether to share my suicidal tendencies with Dr. Ferguson, I couldn't reconcile how medications designed to treat my symptoms also came with the risk of exacerbating them. She warned me of additional side effects like nausea, tiredness, changes in appetite, and excessive thirst. I felt myself become hesitant as I watched Dr. Ferguson pull out a pad from her tailored jacket pocket to write a prescription for Doxepin. I worried about what additional side effects would come, but I was desperate to get better and promised myself I'd continue taking my drugs as prescribed. Before I could admit my anxieties, Dr. Ferguson scheduled our next two-week follow-up and led me out the door.

After the appointment, I drove to Krispy Kreme and ordered half a dozen glazed donuts. Back when my biggest problem was memorizing verses for Sunday school, my dad would take me to the shop as a way to keep me encouraged. We used to stand together and stare behind a large window as the round-shaped pieces of dough sped through the conveyor belt coating each donut with frosting. While I waited for my local CVS to fill my prescription, I licked glaze off my fingers in the Krispy Kreme parking lot and played worship music by David Crowder Band and Jon Foreman. Songs like "Your Love Is Strong" and "You're Everything" soothed my anxious spirit. I tapped my fingers to the beat of the drums and rocked my head from side to side as if I was standing at a worship concert.

In the car, I hypothesized that if I kept praying and reading scripture to build my life around God and prove my piety, he would heal me through Dr. Ferguson. Finally, the pharmacy called to let me know that my prescription was ready. As the pharmacist handed me my new medications at CVS on Lewisville Clemmons Road, I became self-conscious about the six donuts I inhaled and grabbed a vanilla protein bar that Dr. Ferguson would approve of.

* * *

Two weeks into following the new treatment regimen each day as prescribed, I arrived early to my appointment to take advantage of the electric kettle and herbal tea that Dr. Ferguson kept in her waiting room. I was lucky to claim a larger mug before the pack of lunch-hour patients arrived. I picked a bag of chamomile because the box promised to provide calmness and peace. My tea made the room smell like the essential oils aisle at Whole Foods. I removed a grocery receipt from my purse and surveyed the rows of empty chairs around me for mundane details worth recording to create a poem. My idea felt brilliant, like I was creating a potential literary masterpiece. I tried to construct a unique simile to describe the gaudy floral artwork mounted in golden frames that gave the appearance of hotel art. But suddenly, I became distracted by the miniature water fountain with an angel statue that stood on top of a stack of pebbles, which seemed at the time to have spiritual meaning. The trickling noise was supposed to be relaxing, but to me it just sounded like someone using the bathroom. My racing thoughts were difficult to track, a possible symptom of the mania Dr. Ferguson had warned me about. At the same time, I didn't know if I was just being creative and spontaneous, key traits of my personality. I leaned my head against the beige-painted wall and stared at the ceiling, counting the tiles in an attempt to slow down my mind.

For people living with bipolar disorder, a single thought can turn into obsession. Racing thoughts are a common symptom of mania. Rapid thoughts become repetitive, sometimes moving from subject to subject, almost out of nowhere. What stands out for those with bipolar disorder is that these thoughts are unceasing and every coping skill imaginable, like breathing exercises or long walks, fail to provide an end. You become trapped in your own mind.

To distract myself from my thoughts, I looked through a travel magazine that was lying on a side table next to a glass bowl of organic mints. As I flipped through the glossy pages filled with Indian recipes, I was struck by sudden inspiration. On my grocery receipt, I wrote down the names of all the spices listed on those pages, because I believed that knowing these spices was the key to my future happiness. I stopped on a short blurb about the health benefits of turmeric. Ideas kept coming to me—so many dishes to create! I made a list of meals I was going to make my parents at home. Yes, it was true, I was not a good cook at the time, but that was all about to change. Chicken biryani. Chana masala. Samosas. These seemed like the answers I had been looking for.

I kept flipping. Black-and-white photos of the streets of New Delhi felt like a divine revelation. I knew then what I must do: go to India to tell the people about Jesus. I closed my eyes, imagining myself wandering around the markets of Mumbai, picking out different spices and fabrics while befriending the locals. Fifteen minutes in the waiting room was enough to convince me that God wanted me to become a missionary and that he wanted me to cook dozens of Indian dishes.

When Dr. Ferguson appeared in the doorway, she motioned me to her office and handed me yet another chart to rate my moods and symptoms. Whereas in the last visit, I circled all my symptoms four, this time I circled zero for racing thoughts, anxiety, lack of sleep, depression, thoughts of death, and decreased motivation.

Noting the progress on paper, Dr. Ferguson smiled. To her, my answers to the questionnaire signaled that my medications were doing their job, so she kept them the same. Fearing that she'd up the dosages on my medications or change them altogether, I kept my epiphany about traveling to India as a missionary to myself. Her bright red fingernails lacked any imperfections, and I thought about how the smallest details were accounted for in the ways I wanted for myself. I pulled my sweater sleeves over my hands to hide where I picked the skin around my fingers. Dr. Ferguson said that she would see me in a month before congratulating me on my progress.

That night, instead of sleeping, I spent hours watching

different videos of Holi festivals. Inspired, I signed up to volunteer with an organization that rehabilitated human trafficking victims in Mumbai. The next morning, I grabbed random items of clothing from my closet and brought them to a local consignment shop, where I received five hundred dollars and used the money for a nonrefundable deposit toward my housing to secure my spot on the summer volunteer team. During our next appointment, I told Dr. Ferguson about my trip. In response, she replaced the back issues of *National Geographic* with magazines about the stock market and current fashion trends. (She never actually mentioned this to me.) During our monthly follow-up, she said, "I think we need to take you off Doxepin. Clearly it's not a good fit for you."

Frustrated that she did not pick up on the signs earlier with me, I watched as she rubbed her temples. She wrote a prescription for 300 milligrams of Trileptal, a medication originally used for seizures but now also as a mood stabilizer for bipolar disorder. The drug is known to help prevent manic episodes but also comes with side effects like lack of balance, hives, uncontrolled eye movement, and thoughts of suicide. Dr. Ferguson wanted to see if the Trileptal could do what the Doxepin had not: keep me from becoming manic. In the parking lot that day, I emailed the organization in India and said that I had a medical emergency preventing me from visiting. Despite the time difference, the organization's founder responded within minutes. "We're praying for your recovery," he wrote.

* * *

Reflecting on my impulsive decision to pay a five-hundred-dollar nonrefundable deposit on a trip I was no longer taking, I thought about the story of Moses. He was a prophet born to Israelite parents enslaved by the Egyptians. The books of Exodus, Leviticus, Deuteronomy, and Numbers tell the story of how Moses became a prophet and leader who helped save the Israelites from oppression. In the book of Exodus, Moses takes care of his father-in-law's livestock. One day while he is watching over the flock, an angel of the Lord appears to him in a flame out of a bush. He notices at once how the bush is on fire but not burned up. God calls his name from the bush, commanding him to remove his sandals because he is standing on holy ground. Moses hides his face because he is afraid to look at God. The Lord tells him that he has witnessed the misery of the Israelites and expresses his desire to deliver them from the bondage of slavery. He tells Moses he must go to the Pharaoh and bring the Israelites out of Egypt. God and Moses continue to speak while Moses talks through hypothetical situations, like what might happen if the Israelites do not believe that he will deliver them from Egypt. God instructs Moses to throw the staff that he is holding onto the ground. At that moment, the staff turns into a snake. God continues to show him more signs, but Moses doubts his own abilities, complaining that he is slow to speak. God instructs him to take his staff and return to Egypt.

Moses returns to Egypt and begs the Pharaoh to free his people. After the Pharaoh refuses, God brings about a series of plagues on the Egyptian people: water in the Nile River turns to blood, frogs swarm the land, lice fly throughout

Egypt, flies take over the land, livestock die, people break out into boils all over their bodies, large pieces of hail cause destruction, swarms of locusts kill crops, darkness lasts for three days, and, finally, every firstborn son in the land of Egypt is killed, including the Pharaoh's. In grief, the Pharaoh responds to the death of his son by telling the Israelites that they are free to leave. As Moses is leading the Israelites out of Egypt, the Pharaoh changes his mind and sends an army after them. The Israelites reach the Red Sea and fear being trapped as the army comes upon them. But then God instructs Moses to lift his staff, causing the Red Sea to part. The Israelites make it to the other side while the sea closes upon the soldiers, drowning them. In the new land, the wilderness of Sinai, God provides the Israelites with food from the sky and Moses creates water by striking his staff on the rocks. After three months of travel, they reach Mount Sinai. Thunder, lightning, and a thick cloud appear with the voice of a loud trumpet, causing the people to tremble. The Israelites surround the base of the mountain, waiting to see what happens after God forbids them from climbing Sinai. On the mountain, surrounded by smoke, God descends with fire, causing the mountain to shake, and summons Moses. On top of the mountain, God speaks the Ten Commandments to Moses, a set of biblical principles used by Christians and Jews throughout history to shape their moral frameworks. They were taped on the walls of many of my Sunday school classrooms with rules decreeing not to lie or steal. Moses stays on the mountain communing with God for forty days and forty nights. In the end, God gives Moses two tablets of stone with the commandments written by the Lord himself to deliver and teach to the Israelites about living a godly life.

As I read through Exodus after my manic episode, seeing the burning bush, receiving the Ten Commandments, and parting the Red Sea seemed like instances of auditory hallucinations or delusions or even hypomania, like what I experienced in my own life. I thought of Moses speaking to the burning bush and witnessing his staff turn into a snake. Did he experience God, or was he hallucinating? I imagined myself watching Moses from Mount Sinai, surrounded by Israelites, questioning the sanity of their leader for saying that God had given him handwritten rules engraved on pieces of stone. Did he really receive the commandments from God, or had he lost his mind?

I did not know why attempting to diagnose Moses mattered to me then, but in reflecting, I see that I wanted definite answers about whether my decision to spend that five hundred dollars was an expression of my faith or a symptom of my illness. That the answer might be both didn't occur to me then. During my manic episodes, an unclear line existed between delusion and belief. But, in the unknowing—maybe this is where faith exists. For me, the story of Moses became a comfort to believe that insight can possibly exist alongside insanity and that God is present in all things.

* * *

Weeks after the manic episode, I made the decision to reenroll at my college in January 2012, after my friends told me how much they missed having me on campus. Numerous gaps existed from my semester at home. As I watched my friends continue pursuing careers with perceivable ease, every minute I spent struggling to get out of bed felt like further proof that my diagnosis was divine punishment. The hardest part of my diagnosis was not the symptoms themselves, but the overwhelming anxiety that I was wasting my life. More than anything, I wanted to feel like I was making progress.

The morning of move-in day, I removed pieces of clothing from the white hangers in my home closet until they created a pile as tall as the ones I made with dead leaves in my backyard. Without bothering to fold them, I threw the clothes into blue plastic containers.

As I passed through the living room, I saw my mom resting her feet on the leather recliner while finishing her morning devotions. Looking up from her Bible, she removed her reading glasses, formulating what to say.

"If you're not ready to go back to school, we will support whatever you need."

Before packing up the car, I offered a simple nod. I was still working with Dr. Ferguson and taking my medications as prescribed and thought that was enough for me to handle college again. When my parents arrived on campus with me, we appeared to be the only ones there as the city recovered from a snowstorm that left barely two inches of snow on the ground. But in Winston-Salem, that was enough to shut down the entire city. Many businesses stayed closed for the day. Normally while walking down the cobblestone roads of Winston, you can buy pastries baked in a wood-fired brick oven or Moravian stars to hang on your front porch. But that day, the lights in each store were shut off and the sidewalks were abandoned. Large gardens normally filled with fresh vegetables and blooming flowers sold at the weekly farmers market were replaced by dry land that appeared frozen. The mix of snow and salt that covered the roads had the consistency of slush.

Arriving at my room, in the dorm called Gramley Hall, my dad rushed to a corner and waved his hand to remove cobwebs before rolling up the vinyl shade that covered my window. Many girls on campus claimed that Gramley Hall was haunted. The legend went that a girl took her own life by hanging herself on the top floor where I lived. Girls reportedly heard the ghost move furniture in the middle of the night.

My mom still recalls mundane details from that afternoon, like how my body posture changed as soon as we arrived on campus; about how, even without knowing why I was crying, I fought back tears. Part of me hoped that returning to college would be enough to return to my old life. But being back on campus, I suspected that I was not the same person.

Later that afternoon, as I walked alone across the brick sidewalks, I associated the campus with my last memories of being stable, when I felt control over my thoughts and actions. I looked around for other students outside, but I was the only one braving the freezing temperatures. The brick academic buildings with large pillars remained empty, but lights came from windows of the dormitories. My life seemed to have a clear before and after. In my before life, I was happy, social, and able to see the positives in life. Now I could barely get out of bed and felt hopeless and filled with anxiety and often failed to come up with a satisfactory list of reasons to stay alive. Professors complained about my lack of engagement. I buried my hands in my pockets and walked toward the graveyard where my ex, Hunter, and I used to walk through after midnight. This was a place that used to give me comfort while being with him. I could make out the shapes of the tombstones from the sidewalk but turned around before I even arrived. The pain of losing him hit me as I stood alone on the sidewalk, across from the outdoor amphitheater where graduation took place each spring. My gut reaction was that I needed to leave the campus as soon as I could. When I returned from my walk, my phone had several missed calls from friends on campus who wanted to hang out. They left confused voicemails, wondering where I was and wanting to celebrate the start of a new year. I left each message unanswered, unsure of how to explain what was going on with me.

After repacking my car on the same day that I moved in, I placed my room key on the dean's doorstep while the streets were empty. When I arrived back home four hours after they dropped me off, I found my parents watching a Lifetime movie on the couch.

"I need to leave this town. I can't stay here," I told them, holding boxes of my clothes.

Out of solutions, my parents exchanged looks, and I took a seat on the leather couch next to my dad, grabbing one of my mom's famous chocolate chip cookies as we watched the movie in silence.

Chapter 4

A month after I told my parents I needed to move out, I found two roommates on Craigslist looking for someone to rent their extra bedroom in Raleigh, two hours away from Winston-Salem. The city's population almost reaches half a million, nearly twice the population of my hometown. My only frame of reference for Raleigh was that I went there to see concerts of bands like Death Cab for Cutie and Bon Iver at large outdoor venues. My dad also drove me to the state history museum in elementary school to see Abraham Lincoln's presidential portrait.

Before agreeing to move, I drove to see the apartment. The pair of roommates, sisters named Millie and Elise, opened the door and invited me in. Their sixty-pound golden lab bolted from behind them and jumped on me, almost knocking me to the floor. The first thing I noticed about that apartment was its overwhelming blandness—bare walls that blended in with the beige carpet and the bathroom floor that looked like porcelain tile. Back home, I was used to my fuchsia dining room and my lime green kitchen and my basement, where every wall was painted a different color; I was used to the vases and flowers and antique items with which my mom routinely adorned our home. Was it possible that I was already homesick for these things and those colors? Here, at Millie and Elise's place, the only decorations to be found—the only sign that people lived here at all—were wine bottles sitting on the kitchen counter that had been stuffed with Christmas lights. I felt ill, but still desperate to connect.

"I really like what you've done with the place," I said.

The younger sister, Elise, walked me upstairs to show me where my bedroom would be. I stepped over piles of clothes sprawled on the hallway floor next to the laundry machine. The room was half the size of my room at home and had a small window that looked out over the parking lot.

"So what brings you to Raleigh?" she asked.

"I'm just looking for a change."

Struggling to continue having a conversation with me, she put her hands in the back of her jean pockets. Before leaving, I signed the lease.

Prone to making meaning out of every instance, to searching for signs and validation among uncertainty that I was following the precise path that God wanted for my life, I noticed that the house was located on the aptly named Renewal Drive. In my journal that night, I wrote that the street name was a sign from God.

Later that week, I enrolled at North Carolina State University for the spring semester as a non-degree-seeking student. My parents had contributed to a savings account for my college since I was born and offered to continue covering the cost like they had for my freshman year. Since I was now attending a public university, the tuition was much cheaper. I took just a few classes to ease back into school instead of taking on a full course load. Overwhelmed with the large variety of class options compared to my small school, I signed up for what sounded most interesting: Introduction to Companion Animals, Introduction to World Archeology, and American Literature.

On my first day of classes in January, I arrived an hour early to walk around campus. Back home, tedious details like navigating campus and finding the correct buildings were never things that I thought about because every class was three minutes from my doorstep. I felt homesick.

By the time I reached the correct lecture hall for my first class, I heard the professor introducing himself to the students. An entire auditorium filled with about one hundred students faced me as I walked inside.

"Glad to see that you decided to make it to class," the professor said.

Several of the students snickered. The professor waited for me to sit down before he proceeded to speak. When he dismissed class, I was the first to sprint out the door. Luckily for me, my next class, Introduction to Companion Animals, met across the street. I took a seat in the back row, where I watched different groups of friends arrive together and check their phones. When the professor walked in with a leather briefcase covered with PETA stickers, I noticed how she didn't ask for introductions or our names like professors did at my smaller college. I looked for a point of connection on my first day, for a professor to express interest in my life and belief that I could succeed. I barely kept up with my second class of the day because our professor spoke so quickly. She paced around the front of the room with her hands behind her back and said, "You are allowed to bring your pets to class whenever you'd like." I studied her screen-printed shirt with a gigantic husky that she wore beneath a blazer. I looked around the room and imagined several mutts chasing one another during future lectures as our professor spoke about the ethics of dog breeding. How was I going to stay focused? The students around me whispered excitedly about bringing their pets with them. A boy sitting in the front row raised his hand and asked, "Can I bring my rabbit?"

"Yes, of course!"

All I could think about was a larger dog in class eating his rabbit for breakfast, leaving only traces of blood on the carpet.

When I returned to the apartment that afternoon, my roommates had their friends over with snacks spread across the coffee table. While shoving a handful of popcorn in her mouth, Elise looked over from the couch.

"How was your first day?"

I faked a smile, walking myself to my room without introducing myself to anyone there. "Good."

A 2007 study published by *Current Opinion in Psychiatry* found that 75 percent of those who will have a mental health disorder have their onset by the age of twenty-five years old. This means that many, like me, are dealing with symptoms during college years, a time of life when, ideally, you're supposed to be focused on the promising life ahead of you. But when you get sick at such a young age, you are robbed of thinking much about the future, and instead you have to focus on how to survive each day. It became easy for me to believe that the best years of my life were already over. Doctors could not give me any assurances about the quality of life I could expect. They couldn't tell me if I'd ever graduate college, hold a job, get married—anything that seemed worthwhile. When I looked at my peers, I saw people pursuing their dreams, making lifelong friends, doing what people their age are supposed to do. I simply couldn't relate. I felt frozen in time. When I did contemplate the future, all I foresaw was a series of health roadblocks that I'd be lucky to survive.

* * *

Transferring to a school with forty times as many students as where I came from was a change that I never embraced. But I believed that was where God wanted me to be—in Raleigh, at that school—and so I assumed that everything would fall into place. It turns out that that belief has no basis in scripture. I compared myself to Paul, the disciple most known for being the author of thirteen books of the Bible; Timothy, the disciple who accompanied Paul on many missionary journeys to help churches; and John, known as the youngest apostle. Like me, each of them centered their lives around understanding and learning from the ministry of Jesus. I looked up to each one of them as heroes, hoping to obtain the dedication that they showed for their faith throughout their lives.

One year for Christmas, my mother gifted me a silver necklace with a glass pendant that contained a mustard seed, no bigger than a grain of rice. I knew upon ripping off the snowman-patterned wrapping paper that the gift from her was a reference to Jesus saying in the book of Matthew that if you have faith as small as a mustard seed, you can move a mountain.

Jesus says these words after a distressed man comes to him, seeking help for his son, who is possessed by a demon. The father watches in desperation as his son experiences seizures and remains in constant suffering. He describes the possession as causing him to fall into water and fire. At first, he had brought his son to Christ's disciples, but they were unable to cure him. Jesus rebukes the demon, and the boy is cured instantly. The disciples go to Jesus and ask why they could not cure the boy. Jesus tells them because of their lack of faith and says they only need to have faith the size of a mustard seed. Maybe the disciples did not believe Jesus when he gave his closest friends the ability to heal in order to show the glory of God. Maybe they saw the boy's struggles and thought even God could not save him. Jesus says that his closest friends only need to have the amount of faith of the smallest seed that looks like a grain of rice. This seems improbable when coming from a world where I weighed individual choices around what could increase my faith.

The idea of having a faith that felt certain seemed like the entire purpose of life. While my mom was throwing away scraps of wrapping paper that Christmas morning, I snuck the mustard seed necklace into the trash can. I wanted a faith much larger than a mustard seed. I wanted a faith as large as a deeply rooted oak tree, the kind where you had to lean back to see the highest branches in the sky.

* * *

A few days after classes began, I attended a small Christian group gathering. Common in Christian communities, small groups consisting of a few individuals meeting to learn about God are found throughout scripture. The books of Luke, Matthew, and Mark tell the stories of Jesus selecting a small group of twelve men—Peter, James, John, Andrew, Philip, Bartholomew, Matthew, Thomas, James, Thaddaeus, Simon, and Judas—who serve as his community. As I was growing up, pastors said that Jesus modeled modern-day small-group ministry through his disciples, whom he trained to take over his ministry and spread the message of Christianity. Small groups in churches today meet to pray for one another and study scripture. These groups are used to create long-term community and accountability to live a life for God.

I found a group through Campus Crusade for Christ, a college ministry organization that serves thousands of college campuses worldwide, and emailed them about joining. Upon my arrival, I found several girls sitting in a semicircle on the living room floor. Shane & Shane, a Christian band, familiar to me from my youth, played from a pair of portable speakers. As if she were evaluating my outfit, one of the leaders scanned me head to toe with envy.

"How did you get so skinny? Are you on a low-carb diet? I've tried that, but it didn't work for me."

I shook my head. "No, this is just how I look," I replied.

She laughed and said, "So, it must be genetic."

I didn't have the guts to admit that one of the side effects of Cymbalta was loss of appetite. I wanted to say, "My shrinking body is a metaphor for my emotional state." But then

I thought that might sound melodramatic. I grabbed three brownies to signal that I was in fact not dieting. She sat next to me and reached out her hand.

"I'm Allison."

I eyed her "What Would Jesus Do?" bracelets. When she saw me looking, she took a green one off her wrist and handed it to me.

"These are a great way to tell people about Jesus," she said.

At that point, a girl wearing a tan fedora tapped her fork against her glass of water, as if to make a toast. "Tonight," she said, "we're going to discuss the meaning of suffering!"

She reminded me of who I used to be, which made her intolerable. I noticed how she had not stopped smiling since I had arrived and turned every conversation into a discussion about God. Before the group even discussed the topic, I started crying.

"I struggle with depression," I said. "This is a hard thing for me to talk about." The choice to say "depression" instead of "bipolar disorder" was purposeful. I knew from conversations back home that people associated bipolar disorder with extreme mood swings. This wasn't true for me, and I didn't want people thinking it was.

Allison, sitting next to me, cleared her throat.

"Anna, I think that God is calling me to share a scripture with you."

Tossing her waist-long strawberry blonde hair over her shoulder to bow her head, Allison closed her eyes and quoted a verse about heaven from the book of Revelation: "He will wipe away every tear from their eyes. There will be no more death or mourning or crying or pain, for the old order of things has passed away." (21:4). The author of the book of Revelation describes a vision from God of New Jerusalem, a holy city, coming down out of the heavens. He writes that God desires for men to be in fellowship and unity together in this city after death. The New Jerusalem, meaning heaven, is distinguished from what we have on earth by its lack of any pain, sin, or darkness.

Growing up, I had sung worship songs inspired by this verse, songs designed to reassure congregants that one day our suffering would end. Heaven provided us a far-off reality and distant future to strive for, a reality where pain no longer existed. Back before my diagnosis, I spent a lot of time day-dreaming about what eternity with God would look like. But now mental health difficulties kept me firmly in the here and now, on this plane, where suffering was very real and impossible to ignore.

The girls around me in the Bible study said, "Amen" when Allison finished praying, as if she had said something profound. I remained silent. These girls all looked the same to me at that moment. Their outfits perfectly hid the existence of their curves just as churches had taught us to do. They had long hair lightened by the sun from monthlong mission trips in third-world countries. Each of them smelled like a vanilla candle that you might buy your mom as a last-minute Mother's Day gift. I looked around and noticed that each of us was wearing a purity ring on our left ring finger. As a small act of rebellion, I grabbed my ring and stuffed it in my jean pocket. I wasn't like them.

"That's not helpful at all," I told Allison.

"Well God just told me that you needed to hear that," she replied.

I kept eating the brownies on my plate and staring at the clock. Meanwhile the group discussion continued all around me.

As someone fighting to stay alive and taking medications to prevent thoughts of death, I couldn't take solace in the afterlife. Her response reminded me of the many acquaintances who tried to comfort me during periods of depression with affirming, relentlessly positive words.

I did believe that God often spoke through people. But the idea that spirituality had to be uplifting made me question the depth of my own faith. I needed someone to tell me that despair was also a function of faith, that even Jesus wept.

* * *

When Jesus and his disciples travel to Jerusalem for Passover, a holiday commemorating the Israelites' escape from Egypt, they discover when they walk into the courtyard of the temple that the area is filled with tables of money changers and merchants selling livestock. Witnessing the place of worship transformed into a shopping mall, Jesus approaches the money changers' tables and lifts his hands, pours out the coins, flips their tables, and tells the people that the house of prayer had been turned into a den of thieves. The point of this story is typically taken to be the sacred nature of the temple. In my community, Jesus's explosive anger was usually overlooked. Anger, after all, was supposed to be sinful.

But Jesus shows us that anger can sometimes be an appropriate, even righteous response to the world's injustice. Sometimes it's okay to sit with our pain, with our anger. Sitting with these girls, I was angry that the Bible was being used as a weapon designed to minimize my experience. Surely that wasn't what a loving God would do. I imagined myself with Jesus, flipping over their coffee tables and scattering the empty plates and brownie crumbs.

* * *

In the days that followed, Allison reached out to grab lattes. Desperate to make friends, I regarded her invitation as a sign from God that I had found a friend group where I belonged—or maybe that I needed to apologize for snapping at her during Bible study. In hopes of covering the dark circles underneath my eyes and the acne caused by my medication, a side effect of the Lamictal, I took twenty minutes to apply concealer before meeting her.

When Allison saw me from across the coffee shop, she ran over, embracing me in an awkward side hug. Hoping that walking around might make the conversation less awkward, I suggested we get our drinks to go. We walked the brick sidewalks and passed by other students roaming down Hillsborough Street when Allison asked my major and what brought me to NC State. I didn't trust her enough to go into the backstory of how I ended up there, so I deflected.

"What are you studying?" I asked.

"I'm studying Spanish. I'm planning to be a missionary after I graduate."

I kept asking questions about her life, determined to keep the focus off me. She eventually interrupted, saying, "How have you been seeing God at work in your own life?"

We sat on a bench, and I looked straight ahead at an oak tree, beneath which sat a group of students.

"I'm not sure," I said.

"Are you reading your Bible?"

I lied. "Yes, I do that every day."

Though spending time with God for me had always meant reading through scripture and meditating on the words of God, whenever I opened my Bible while living in Raleigh, I struggled to pay attention to more than a paragraph.

She took a sip of her latte and put on a pair of oversize sunglasses bigger than her face as we sat on a bench outside one of the engineering buildings.

"What about praying? Maybe your depression would subside if you asked for more help."

Her suggestion made me want to cry.

"Yes, I've tried that, too."

Again, I was lying to her. I did not know how to say to her, to my friends, to God, that I no longer understood the purpose of prayer. Depression took away my motivation to close my eyes and clasp my hands like I once did. I had spent most of my life offering prayers of gratitude, begging for forgiveness from God, listing off sins in a journal I kept underneath my pillow. I cried out to be healed for months after my diagnosis while driving my car to psychiatry and therapist appointments. The more time that passed, the less likely that seemed. I lacked any words for God. Where to begin?

She crossed her arms and looked out into the distance, trying to formulate other quick fixes that might relieve my suffering. Prayer, time in scripture, and poorly written books authored by pastors were the most common salves to any hardship offered by those in my community—including me. It seemed that what I was suffering from had stumped Allison, making her unsure of what else to offer, so we sat in silence. I tried to think of some common ground. I remembered just in time that she had mentioned in Bible study that she enjoyed books.

"Are you reading anything good right now?" I asked.

She took off her sunglasses and looked over at me before putting her hand on my thigh, causing me to scoot farther away from her.

"Have you heard of *Praying for Your Future Husband: Preparing Your Heart for His*?"

The title alone made me want to run, but I stayed still instead, listening to her talk through her desire to find someone and get married right out of college. This confirmed to me that we were on different playing fields. Marriage was the furthest thing from my mind. For every guy interested in dating me, there was an assortment of questions about my life that I refused to answer. Since my diagnosis, I had convinced myself that it was impossible to meet anyone willing to settle down with me. But still, I sat there listening to her talk to me about her endless prayers to find a godly husband, something I thought would never be mine. She said, "Can you pray that I don't struggle with loneliness while I'm single?"

I tried to imagine any point in my life where that was not

an emotion lingering in the back of my mind. "No. Everyone is lonely."

She studied my face, trying to see if this was some kind of joke.

Before leaving, Allison gave me a hug and held me for a moment before putting her hand on my shoulder.

"Before we leave, can I pray for God to give you joy?"

It was not unusual behavior for Christians in my community to pray for me about my struggles, whether in youth group or in public spaces like coffee shops. But this time, I picked up her hand and placed it by her side before shaking my head. I knew when she walked away that that was the last I'd see of her.

Chapter 5

When I started classes in Raleigh, I had two psychiatrists: Dr. Ferguson, and then Dr. Guinn, whom Dr. Ferguson had referred me to. Dr. Guinn had told me that I needed to find friends, but I found that difficult to do while managing my depression symptoms. I decided I also wanted a Christian therapist, someone who could help me learn some new coping skills. Throughout my therapist search, my parents insisted on covering the costs. After some Google searches, I discovered Whitney. Her home page included quotes from Christian authors like Henri Nouwen and Thomas Merton, whose words had provided me comfort in the past. Her biography section featured photos of her walking downtown in a leather jacket that matched her dark curly hair. This was much different than the staged photos on other sites that looked like the therapist's portraits belonged in outdated church directories. Under hobbies, she listed going to the local art museum, visiting coffee shops, the state farmers market, and concerts. She appeared like someone who would be my friend. I sent her an email to make an appointment. She followed up within an hour, saying she could see me the next afternoon.

Whitney's office was on the edge of downtown back before

high-rise apartments and hotels pervaded the skyline. Opening Whitney's door, I found a fridge in the waiting room filled with practically the only thing that I drank: Diet Coke. One of my favorite bands, Arcade Fire, played from the speakers. Not one for small talk, she jumped right in.

"What is one thing that you like about yourself?"

I was shocked by the question; self-love, I thought, was nothing more than vanity.

"Well," I said, "I've always thought that I have a cool last name that would look good on the back of a jersey."

"Seriously, though, you can't think of anything else?"

Taking a few minutes to reflect, all I could think about was my long list of recent failures.

"I've always seen myself as a sinner in need of grace, which I've interpreted to mean that I'm not supposed to like anything about myself."

"But what about the part of scripture where God tells us to love ourselves?"

"Where did you come up with that?"

When Jesus is questioned about the greatest commandment, he says to love God, but he doesn't stop there. His second commandment is to love yourself as much as you love your neighbor. This is from a verse in the book of Matthew that I'd memorized at an early age, but I'd never paid attention to the part about loving myself; that part of the verse was never discussed in sermons. I became so wrapped up in my identity as a sinner, unworthy of everything in my life, that I failed to see myself as worthy of love.

"I want you to go through your Bible and mark passages

that speak of God's love for people," she said. "I know that doesn't exactly sound like fun, but I think it might help you."

Before I left, she tossed me a Diet Coke and told me to see her the following week.

I waited until I was sitting in the parking lot before our next appointment to do the assignment. I found the idea of loving myself too uncomfortable; I put it off until the last possible moment. I could not see how self-love and the sin of selfishness were different from each other. I opened my Bible to the first page in the book of Genesis, filled with scripture describing the creation of the world. I got to the part about God creating humankind and felt caught off guard: "So God created mankind in his own image, in the image of God he created them; male and female he created them." Reading this verse, I was struck by how it described the ways in which human beings are reflections of the divine nature and how the characteristics of a holy God dwell in each of us. It seemed to counter everything I'd been taught before about how human beings are depraved and unworthy of love. I'd encountered these verses before, but I had never noticed this insight until now.

As I lay on Whitney's L-shaped couch, I told her about that verse and its effect on me. She pulled a Bible off her bookshelf and stood up, as though she were giving a sermon. She opened it to a page in the book of Romans, written by the Apostle Paul, and read aloud: "For I am convinced that neither death nor life, neither angels nor demons, neither the present nor the future, nor any powers, neither height nor depth, nor anything else in all creation, will be able to separate us from the love of God that is in Christ Jesus our Lord." Paul wrote this book as a letter of encouragement to Christians in Rome, who were a mix of Gentiles and Jews, and many of whom were illiterate slaves. In the passage Whitney chose, Paul recognizes the love of God as foundational to what it means to live a life of faith. As I listened to Whitney read the scripture, it was as though Paul were speaking directly to me.

Whitney shut the Bible and placed it back on the shelf next to her psychiatry textbooks and didn't say anything else. A wave of peace rushed over me. My view of myself didn't suddenly change. I still wasn't sure how I could love myself. But that was the moment when I clearly heard, for the first time, God telling me that I was enough.

* * *

Whitney and I continued to meet throughout the semester — for one hour, once a week, and then eventually increasing to twice a week when my depressive symptoms persisted.

Her emphasis on self-love gradually changed how I treated my body. She taught me to think of my body as a temple deserving of respect. I started eating healthier. I took her suggestion to start exercising, which she thought might help improve my mood. I started running. Each of my most vivid memories in Raleigh involves running right before sunset.

I trashed all my baggy clothes designed to make me look almost invisible and went vintage shopping, picking out clothing that felt more like me. Before my diagnosis, I wore bright colors; after my diagnosis, I wore only earth tones. My closet became several different shades of gray. With Whitney's help, I learned to reconnect with these wants and desires without fearing that I was being selfish and therefore rebelling against God. And, even with all this progress, Whitney stayed persistent in encouraging me to get more involved in the community.

One Sunday, three months after my sessions with Whitney began, I visited a nondenominational church that met inside an old Coca-Cola warehouse. The pastor, Phillip, was well-known and had spoken at Christian conferences that I'd attended when I was younger.

In modern evangelical churches, pastors can come to be seen as something akin to celebrities. Lacking any governing boards or form of oversight, nondenominational churches are often built around, and made in the image of, particular pastors. When I was growing up, I believed the pastors at my churches had VIP access to God. Everyone wanted to have them over for dinner, to have coffee with them, to be part of their circles. All this attention, I believe, contributed to what I now see as narcissism.

Every church that I attended throughout my childhood and early adulthood was part of the Gospel Coalition, an active organization of thousands of churches across denominations that sought to apply scripture to culture, current events, and issues in daily life. What set them apart was that their teachings looked at these issues through a narrow lens, dismissing other theological interpretations of engaging with the world as wrong and heretical. I actively read their blog posts, which were written by pastors and scholars I followed, including Mark Driscoll, John Piper, and D. A. Carson.

When I walked inside the church in Raleigh, a greeter

stood by the door and offered a mechanical smile before handing me a weekly program. This reminded me of the churches that I'd grown up in, but still I felt out of place. Being in a space surrounded by Christians who may or may not view my struggles as sinful made me fight back tears until I finally put on my aviator sunglasses.

The lack of windows and the dark walls in the sanctuary made the room seem like an amphitheater for rock concerts. Aisles of plastic chairs were placed in four separate sections around the center stage. Volunteers used flashlights to guide people to their seats. They waved them as if directing a long line of traffic. When someone directed me to a seat in the front row, I shook my head, but the darkness kept him from noticing. The background music prevented the volunteer from hearing me say that I wanted a seat as far from the stage as possible.

He continued to wave his hand while I stood still in the aisle. Eventually I walked backward and placed my purse beneath a seat in the back row, closest to the exit. I watched as the rows became filled with groups of college students and young families. The row where I sat remained empty until a couple with similar haircuts sat three chairs away from me. Suddenly afraid that they might introduce themselves and ask questions about my life, I opened my Bible and pretended to read. Moving my finger down the crinkled page, I landed on a verse but could not see a single word in the dark. As the church band took the stage, the sound of clicking drumsticks and guitarists tuning their instruments ended the conversations around me.

While swaying back and forth onstage, a woman held her microphone stand and sang the opening verse of Hillsong United's popular song "Healer." The song, written by Australian songwriter Michael Guglielmucci after a terminal cancer diagnosis, had become a source of controversy when it was revealed that Guglielmucci had received no such diagnosis. Instead, he'd fabricated the diagnosis to conceal his addiction to pornography.

> *You walk with me through fire*
> *And heal all my disease.*

A young, bearded college student with an electric keyboard played suspenseful synthesizers that looped like a DJ set list. Although I wanted to leave, I feared what people would think of me if they saw me leaving mid-service. Instead, I walked to the room a few rows away from me with a neon sign that read "Prayer Room." During their prayer, one of the volunteers pressed her hands against the shoulders of a woman who sat on the bare concrete floor. Her whispering prevented me from hearing what she was asking God for. The only other volunteer in the prayer room stood in the doorway and looked close to my dad's age. He peered out into the crowd as if he was predicting who else in the congregation needed prayer.

I assumed that he would approach me and ask for my prayer request, but when I opened my eyes, he was still looking out at the audience, ignoring my presence. A male college student about my age walked in, and the volunteer immediately approached him. I watched the volunteer take off his baseball cap as a sign of respect for the moment of prayer. As I watched them pray together, I remembered how at some churches men felt uncomfortable praying with women who were not their wives. There are many ways to interpret the volunteer's actions, and I will never know his reasoning for not praying with me. But because of where I was in my life, I made the assumption that I had done something wrong. His ignoring me furthered the idea in my mind that men did not feel safe with me. Growing up in my community, I was used to hearing women described as "spiritual stumbling blocks" for distracting men from speaking to God. The term had actually been applied to me, when my college pastor asked me to leave the church in order to keep my ex, Hunter, focused on his faith. His sexual attraction to me was seen as sinful because I was not his wife.

Driving away that afternoon, I knew that this would be the last time that I attended church while living in Raleigh. As much as I wanted to connect, I felt too broken to participate in a community of Christians. At the same time, I was learning to acknowledge the depth of my emotions without judging them or treating them as wrong.

I rehashed the entire incident in my following therapy session with Whitney. I could tell by her face that she wanted to temper her anger.

"This must bring back memories for you of how your college pastor handled you at church, seeing you as a stumbling block," she said before noticing that I was tearing up. "I just hope that you know that none of these behaviors are found in scripture. It's not your fault."

She put my case file filled with notes down onto the coffee table.

"Maybe that's just where you are right now and that's okay."

As I sat there across from her, I wanted to believe that she was right. I had watched friends from high school gradually walk away from their faith upon reaching college, now free of having to face religious obligations under their family's roofs. Sometimes I envied their decisions, the freedom they seemingly found. I understood very well the amount of pain caused by faith communities that helped form my understanding of myself and the world around me. But even that was not enough to get me to walk away, for reasons that I did not understand. Perhaps I was too scared to walk away, to lose what shaped me. Maybe those who left were braver than me. Or maybe this endless search for God among broken systems, the belief that Christ existed beyond the mistakes of people in positions of leadership, maybe that was what it meant to practice faith.

* * *

After midterms in March 2011, my college pastor, Jason, texted to ask me to help him find a birthday gift for his wife. His request felt out of the blue. I had been struggling with depression for months since my breakup with Hunter. At church, I tried to appear put together, but I was still in love with him.

Jason met me outside a furniture store downtown that sold high-end food at the glass front counter. He waved as I approached. As soon as we walked inside, a sales associate approached us about deals on velvet couches, but eventually she picked up that neither of us were interested and walked away. I looked over at Jason as he browsed around the store, clearly deep in thought. I had a feeling that he wanted to talk to me about something important. We approached the display case filled with exotic truffles at the front of the store. He chose the pepper-and-turmeric-flavored chocolate, the least popular ones among locals. As the salesclerk wrapped the chocolates in a brown box, my pastor reported that Hunter had been selected as the church intern. He said, "I think he's a real asset to our church community." I opened my mouth to respond, but nothing came out. We exited the store and began walking toward Jason's church office.

As we walked across the crosswalk by the best coffee shop in town, Jason said, "I'm removing you from the leadership team. I don't want your pain to be a distraction to Hunter's spiritual growth anymore." When I did not respond, he added, "I'm worried about him." I felt completely crushed and angry. I had not shared anything with Jason about my relationship with Hunter other than our breakup.

I wondered if he knew how Hunter insisted on walking with me in graveyards to keep from being seen together in public. I wondered if he knew about how he never introduced me to his friends because he said they'd hate my personality. I wondered if he knew about the times when he told me to change my outfits when I wore a low-cut shirt. But most of all, I wondered if he knew about the nights in the back seat of Hunter's car, where every boundary I set was ignored. Why was I being punished?

As the weeks went on, I tried going to the church services until Jason said that my presence was too much for Hunter, who was still trying to get over me while dating the girl he left me for. Hunter apparently could not stand to be in the same room with me without running away. This only reinforced my feeling that I was a seductress, causing a man I loved to fall away from God.

This line of thought, which punishes women and treats them like potential temptresses, goes all the way back to how those in my community interpret Adam and Eve, the first humans found in the book of Genesis. When Adam and Eve live in the Garden of Eden, God tells them that they can have whatever they want except fruit from the tree of good and evil. He warns them that eating from the tree will result in death. But then a serpent tempts Eve to eat the fruit, and she takes a bite before giving the apple to Adam. Many evangelical men I grew up with saw Eve as a temptress who causes Adam to stumble away from God. The fact that Adam listens to Eve instead of God makes her a hindrance to his relationship with his creator. My religious leaders never addressed Adam's personal responsibility in choosing to listen to Eve.

I've witnessed Christians in my community treat women differently from men for my entire life. This dynamic of prescribed gender roles that I grew up with contradicts the ministry of Jesus. In the synoptic Gospels, each writer gives an account of Jesus going to dinner with a group of Pharisees. A woman known in scripture as a sinner hears that Jesus is in town and arrives with an alabaster flask of expensive ointment. She interrupts the meal and sits at Jesus's feet, weeping as she wets his feet with her tears. One of the disciples responds apathetically and accuses her of wasting the ointment that could have been sold for a large amount and given to the poor. Jesus rebukes them and says that the woman did a beautiful thing for him by washing his feet. Still, the men complain that Jesus allowed a sinner to touch him. Jesus could have shamed and banished her or treated her like how my college youth pastor responded to me or how the man in the prayer room ignored my need for prayer. Instead, Jesus blesses the woman and saves her from her sins. I wanted to be treated by the men in my community the way Jesus treated that woman. The improbability of that kept me from having many deep friendships with Christian men. Dating remained the furthest thing from my mind.

* * *

As I continued meeting with Whitney over the summer following my first completed semester at NC State, she asked me during one of our sessions:

"What are some goals that you can make for your life right now?"

"It feels like there are weeks when the only things I can do are get out of bed and make appointments on time."

"In doing those things, do you recognize that you're accomplishing something?"

I shook my head. Since my diagnosis, I felt like time moved quickly and I wasted every moment trying to get healthy at the expense of not enjoying my college experience. I admitted to Whitney that the only thing that helped me feel less alone was writing down my thoughts, even if half the time what I wrote made no sense. She asked, "Would you feel comfortable reading your writing aloud to me?" I felt conflicted but agreed.

Soon, our appointments revolved around these journal entries and having me write letters to people in my past, like old pastors, to work through my anger. In six months, I filled up five journals, each with fragmented recollections of my own history—specifically the events leading up to my diagnosis. Whenever a memory of that time emerged, I pulled out my journal to write it down.

One afternoon, while I read a paragraph about missing my ex, I noticed Whitney tapping her fingers against her thigh.

"Is examining the past helping you move forward?"

When Whitney asked this, I remembered a story from the book of Genesis. Lot lives in the city of Sodom, known as a place for evil and sin. He refuses to leave regardless of what he witnesses. Scripture does not reveal to us Lot's internal thoughts, nor does it provide reasons for why he stayed. Perhaps he fears what might happen if he flees, or, in spite of the evil he witnesses, Sodom still feels like home. In the verse about the city's destruction, two angels lead Lot and his family away from the city. Lot's wife, who is never named in scripture, chooses to leave her war-torn homeland for a new life with her husband in a peaceful land. But she looks back on their way out of the city. Her desire to remember her homeland results in God turning her into a pillar of salt. She became a memorial, a warning symbol to those like me, prone to ruminate on the past.

Noticing that she wasn't getting through to me, Whitney offered: "Anna, have you spent much time looking at the life of Jesus? Religious institutions never accepted him. Maybe that's where you need to focus."

Before concluding our session, Whitney leaned in against the doorway.

"Promise me that you'll take care of yourself?"

* * *

That night, I opened my Bible and read the story of Christ's temptation. In the synoptic Gospels, John baptizes Jesus in the Jordan River. His baptism symbolizes his decision to give up his life to God, marking the beginning of his ministry on earth. As soon as Jesus emerges from the water, the heavens open. John hears God's voice: "This is my Son, whom I love; with him I am well pleased" (Matthew 3:17). The Holy Spirit overcomes Jesus. Those who witness the baptism leave knowing that Jesus is indeed who he says he is: the son of God. Following the baptism, he goes into the desert for forty days and forty nights to fast. While alone, he is separate from everyone, including the religious elite who question his authority as well as his disciples. During these days, he eats nothing and eventually starves. Satan mocks him and tells him to turn a stone into a loaf of bread, that if he really is the son of God that he claims to be, he could do it. Satan then shows Jesus all the kingdoms in the world and promises that he will give him all the glory if he chooses to worship him. Still, Jesus rejects Satan. What bothered me about this story is that the Bible doesn't provide an inner depiction of how much anguish Jesus feels in these moments of starvation and temptation, or whether he begins to doubt his purpose on earth. This is what I can identify with.

Eventually, Satan leads Jesus to the Holy City and stands with him on the highest point of the temple. He demands that he throw himself down. In the sermons I heard growing up, this event was presented as Satan tempting Jesus to somehow prove himself, to demonstrate his power.

But that night, as I read, I wondered whether Jesus ever thought about taking his own life, whether my obsessive thoughts would have been relatable to him. I felt pestering thoughts about my own death and imagined Satan talking to me the way he talked to Jesus, tempting me to jump. My mind kept circling the idea that if I ended my life, the pain would cease.

Even though I questioned God's presence in my life, I did not doubt that Christ understood the extent of my pain in ways that no one else did. The image of Jesus wandering through the desert alone for forty days while Satan offered quick exit plans mirrored my own loneliness and despair. Pondering this story, I felt relief. For the first time in weeks, I didn't feel like I was alone. I closed my Bible and drifted off to sleep.

* * *

As a way of ridding myself of the past, I set my prayer journals on fire. These journals contained prayers and lists of sins that I had documented throughout high school and college. Whenever I reread the entries, I noticed that the writing was frantic, always driven by fear and anxiety. I didn't want to reread them anymore.

I walked to a nearby pharmacy and purchased a red box of kitchen matches. I gathered the journals stacked underneath my bed and placed them on my balcony. As cars sped by my apartment building, I lit a match and placed it on top of the stack of journals, forgetting to close the door of my apartment, resulting in my kitchen filling with smoke and the fire alarm going off.

The fire was supposed to be redemptive, a way for me to burn away my old understanding of God. I stood in the doorway, watching as my apologies to God turned to ash. I wanted to believe in a God who did not require long lists of every bad thought or action in order to earn his love, but there was a difference between knowing and believing. In my therapy sessions with Whitney, I had started to come to an intellectual understanding of a different conception of God, but, emotionally, I still feared a vindictive God, a God eager to damn me for all eternity.

Even now, these old beliefs continue to shape my thoughts and actions—they are still a part of me. The fire didn't free me; instead, I felt numb. The amount of smoke caused me to pass out.

When I awoke in the morning, I found myself covered with a thick layer of dust, lying beneath the dining room table, which had never been used. I wanted to believe that ritual would mark a new beginning, but I felt no different from the day before. Can any of us ever be truly free from the ideas that shape us? Even those who choose to walk away from faith have an identity formed by renunciation—I'm not convinced that they ever fully rid themselves of the past.

I'd moved to Raleigh seeking escape, but I remained haunted. Sweeping the ashes off the porch, I noticed how the flames had burned a hole through one of the planks of wood—forever marked.

Chapter 6

One month before I set my balcony ablaze, my mom recommended that I apply to smaller schools. My parents noticed from my grades that attending a large university did not appear like a good fit for me. Their commitment to helping me led them to cover the costs of getting me into a college where I belonged. I applied to Hope College in Holland, Michigan, for the spring term of 2013 after a Wikipedia search revealed that my favorite singer, Sufjan Stevens, had briefly attended the Christian school in the mid-nineties. I thought that the college's name symbolized what I needed in my own life. My parents agreed to keep funding my college education as they had with my older sister and believed that Hope might finally be a good fit for me after all.

* * *

It wasn't by accident that I chose to attend a Christian college. After attending a Southern Baptist high school and abiding by its many strict rules, I swore that I'd never go to a Christian college. But attending two non-faith-affiliated schools made me want to try a Christian school. I wanted to take religion classes and learn about theology.

Christian colleges vary widely. Some focus on equipping

students to serve the church. Some Christian colleges ban smoking and drinking, regardless of whether students are of legal age. Some have gender-segregated floors with assigned hours when the opposite sex can visit. Some ban premarital sex, including gay sex. Some, including ones my friends attended, had mandatory chapel attendance.

Some Christian colleges offer all the majors you'd find at a public university while also working faith into the curriculum. Hope falls into this category. Founded in 1851, Hope had grown to accommodate Christians from all different backgrounds. What I liked about Hope was that chapel services and practicing Christianity were not mandatory. I'd be free to participate in faith however I felt comfortable.

* * *

After being accepted and enrolling at Hope, the registrar's office called and emailed me several times because I kept forgetting to sign up for classes online. By the time I did, most of the courses—like International Relations, Religion and Politics, and Philosophy of Law—were filled. Talking to the admission's representative on the phone, I figured I'd major in political science or art.

"Most students transferring focus on fulfilling their general requirements first," she said.

I listened to her name different English, history, and philosophy courses that sounded like recipes for me to fail. Finally, she said, "We do have a slot left in Introduction to Poetry. Dr. Glidsan is one of our students' favorite professors on campus; her classes fill up fast." After spending so much time journaling and writing in Raleigh, poetry felt like an extension of the therapeutic work that I was doing.

* * *

When I first arrived in Holland, Michigan, at Hope College for my first semester, a student-led orientation handed out sheets of blank paper and instructed us to write letters to our future selves about what we wanted to accomplish in college and who we hoped to become. I looked with jealousy at the other students sitting at desks around me, scribbling notes to themselves. The orientation leader collected the notes and promised to mail them to us in five years.

* * *

Dr. Glidsan had already handed out the poetry syllabus to students by the time I found a seat on the first day of classes. The tables were pushed together to form a large rectangle. A blond girl next to me wearing a pantsuit moved over her stack of study materials for the LSAT and smiled at me as I sat down in the empty seat. The girl to my right wore oversize glasses and pulled out a drawing pad filled with impressive pictures of landscapes, which made me want to be her friend. Dr. Glidsan's confident voice and commanding presence jolted me to pay attention. Her thick black hair was held back with a claw clip. She noticed me studying her hair and ran her hands through it.

"I just like to embrace the mess," she said.

While pacing back and forth, she explained that she would teach us a different type of poem each week. Reading through the syllabus, I highlighted words and their listed definitions that were foreign to me, like *pantoum*, *villanelle*, and *sestina*. Villanelles are often used to chronicle a writer's obsessions; needless to say, obsessions were something I was familiar with. Sestinas feature the repetition of end words in the six stanzas, which causes readers to see how complex language can be, something that eventually changed how I approached scripture. I had never learned how to look at and analyze the Bible as a piece of literature filled with literary elements that contained a deeper meaning. What drew me initially to poetry is how poets capture an emotion or moment in time so concretely while also abiding by the framework of each form.

"Every class," Dr. Glidsan said, "I'll provide printouts of the best poems from students for us to review. The best way to learn how to write poetry is to learn from others."

I made it my goal that day to have one of my poems featured by the end of the semester. She sat down in the seat at the front of the room and said, "The class is structured around making your own chapbook. You must turn in yours on the last day of class with at least ten poems. Throughout the semester, I will write notes on your drafts and tell you if it's ready for your chapbook or if you need to keep editing. You can submit as many drafts as you'd like."

For our first assignment, Dr. Glidsan asked us to write a poem using anaphora, which meant utilizing repetition of the same words. With the examples given to us, the repetition could be as simple as a single word or as long as an entire page. She reminded us of something written in the syllabus: we were required to turn in handwritten copies of each of our poems. She believed that writing by hand allowed people to become more creative. Before class was over, I tried to think of a topic to write about. Dr. Glidsan wrapped up her class the way she ended all classes, saying, "Stay up late. Keep the music loud. Make interesting choices."

My first poem that semester was about missing North Carolina—the large portions of food, warm weather, and walking through Reynolda Gardens during the summertime. Though I never felt a strong tie to Southern culture, now that I was gone for the first time, I felt a sense of nostalgia. My long last name and tan skin caused people to ask what country I was from. There was a version of the South defined for me over and over again through seeing the lives of my classmates and friends from church, but it wasn't the only narrative about where I lived. Even if it didn't determine my reasoning to move to Michigan, I hoped that going to my parents' home would help me find a place where I finally fit in.

I made lists in my journal of everything that I missed back home: the ocean breeze of the Outer Banks, climbing trees in the backyard of my childhood home, lattes at Krankies coffee shop, and morning carolers at my college in Winston during Christmastime. Unsure of how everything fit together into a poem, I jotted down more and more memories.

All I knew was that I wanted "home" to be the refrain, for the poem to capture the complexities of calling North Carolina my birthplace while also feeling like an outsider. I handed in the poem and awaited feedback.

During class the following week, Dr. Glidsan handed out the stapled packet of poems by my classmates for us to review.

As soon as I got mine, I searched through each page, looking for my own, but found nothing.

When classes ended, I waited anxiously as Dr. Glidsan handed back our poems with notes. The notes I received contained ideas for major revisions, for me to step away from trying to make readers feel an emotion and instead show them images of North Carolina. I walked back to my room in tears. Upset that I didn't do a good job on the first assignment, I called my mom.

"Anna, it's just one assignment," she said. "Why do you care so much about writing a poem?"

Early on, it became clear that Dr. Glidsan had a magnetic personality. The memoir that she wrote about her childhood was a *New York Times* bestseller. She practiced yoga at the studio downtown and rode her bike across campus. During her office hours, the lobby of the English department practically became her own waiting room. Students formed a line in the hallway to meet with her. All I wanted was her approval.

With every poem, Dr. Glidsan slashed through my words with her favorite purple pen. She said that I focused too much on abstract images, things that could not be perceived by the five senses. I wrote big sweeping statements about fear and love, but she wanted me to focus more on the mundane details of my life—details that still seemed meaningless to me. I was so disconnected from my body that processing my senses was difficult. No one had ever taught me how. But I took her advice and started to fill my poems with the little things I noticed over the course of a day.

Doubting my ability to write poems, I skipped a few classes.

But then Dr. Glidsan started emailing me before class each week, making sure that I was planning to be there.

* * *

While at Hope, I began meeting with a psychiatrist named Dr. Lasko, who managed my medications. When we met for the first time, she told me about her dedication to training for the Boston Marathon. She smelled of sweat and wore her greasy hair pulled back into a ponytail as if she went running before our appointments. I told her about my difficulty focusing and getting my work done. She said, "This has more to do with your ADHD than your bipolar diagnosis." At that point, I still took Vyvanse to manage my symptoms. She pulled out a pad of paper and wrote an additional prescription for Adderall.

"Take this whenever you need a boost," she said. She handed over the piece of paper without any other feedback. The medication comes with the side effects of loss of appetite, insomnia, mood swings, and nausea. Both medications are amphetamines, drugs that activate the central nervous system but can also trigger mania. I took Adderall and Vyvanse as prescribed by Dr. Lasko in addition to the mood stabilizers previously prescribed to me and noticed that I could concentrate more easily. On the downside, I experienced manic episodes every month for the rest of college. The mania felt like a nice break from my depression. Sometimes I stayed up all night writing poems, realizing only in the morning that none of the writing made sense.

* * *

Two months into the semester, I visited Dr. Glidsan in office hours and took a seat across from her, immediately breaking into tears of frustration.

"I want to become a poet," I said.

She threw her hands up in the air.

"You already are one. I think that you should be a creative writing major," she replied.

"But you write revisions on all my poems, and they never get chosen for class."

"I think you can get better," she replied. "That's what I'm here to help you with. You have what it takes to write."

Genuinely taken aback, I said, "I'm not sure what you see in me."

She placed her hand on her chin. "You notice the small details," she said. "You notice things that a lot of people miss or ignore. Those details should be like the best whiskey we keep on a shelf, only to bring out when people come over. When you write your poems, bring out those details. That's you. That's your vision. I want you to write what only you can write."

I sat silently, trying to keep the mascara from flowing down my cheeks. Then she asked, "How do you like it here in Michigan?"

I opened my mouth and, without thinking, told her everything—about my diagnosis, about my chronic feelings of alienation everywhere I went, about not knowing if I belonged in a church community anymore, about my nagging sense of my own unworthiness. When I realized how long I'd been talking, I covered my mouth. "I'm sorry," I said. "I overshared."

She laughed. "Most creative writing professors also double as therapists," she said. "Don't worry."

"I just don't know if I belong here."

"Everybody feels that way. Some people are just better at hiding it. You're going to be okay."

She pulled out a piece of paper and wrote down a list of dates of when poets were going to be doing readings on campus. Then she got up and pulled some books off her shelves and handed them to me. I told her I would attend every poetry reading and read as many of these books as I could. I felt as though these books were the company I needed at the time.

Walking back to my room that day, I thought of all the college representatives who used to visit my high school, assuring us students that our college years would be the best of our lives. I remembered the brochures filled with images of smiling friends hanging out on the quad or eating in a dining hall, and how I used to picture myself in such settings. If my college years up until that point were made into a brochure, it would consist of a series of photographs of me sleeping through classes, walking to a psychiatric appointment, or eating alone at Burger King.

But I could also see that my time at Hope was somehow different. If it wasn't brochure-worthy, it was still meaningful, even beautiful. Moments of grace can be hard to come by, and even when they do come, the feeling can be fleeting. This fact doesn't make such moments any less real or less true. That afternoon, reflecting on my conversation with Dr. Glidsan, was such a moment. After years of searching, I was surprised to discover, in the eyes of my teacher and in the words of those poets, that I'd already been found. That there were things only I could say. That all the little details, the things that mattered most to me, might also matter to God.

* * *

One day in class, Dr. Glidsan told us that we'd be discussing a poem by Elizabeth Bishop titled "One Art." I didn't feel particularly engaged. Donning a black hoodie with the hood pulled up, I rested my head on the desk in front of me.

But then Dr. Glidsan started to read, and the poem's first line got my attention: "The art of losing isn't hard to master."

I felt that I knew something about losing. Even with my newfound sense of purpose at Hope, my life could sometimes feel like a long list of losses—some self-inflicted and some beyond my control—starting from the day of my bipolar diagnosis. I'd lost my sense of myself. I'd lost my belief in the world as a safe place. I'd lost my faith. I'd lost my home. I'd lost friends. I'd lost Hunter. I couldn't imagine a life that didn't include the daily grieving of those losses, a life where I mainly wandered through a sorrowful past.

And yet Bishop was describing loss as an art, and one that could be mastered. Dr. Glidsan kept reading:

> *Practice losing farther, losing faster:*
> *places, and names, and where it was you meant*
> *to travel. None of these will bring you disaster.*

I gasped, and my classmates, startled, looked over at me as I fought back tears. A girl handed me a tissue. I knew about losing places and names. I knew about losing the places I'd meant to travel, losing my vision of where I thought my life would take me.

Bishop ends the poem directly addressing someone she's lost:

> *—Even losing you (the joking voice, a gesture*
> *I love) I shan't have lied. It's evident*
> *the art of losing's not too hard to master*
> *though it may look like (* Write *it!) like disaster.*

Sitting there listening, and later, as I reread "One Art," I came to love Bishop's restraint, the way her art imposes structure on topics that aren't linear. Like Bishop, I wanted grief and abandonment to be easily manageable. Maybe they couldn't be, but poetry had given her, and could give me, a way of living with these losses. Bishop had gotten this exactly right: the losses had come, one after another, but they hadn't brought me disaster. I had my experience, and it was mine, and no one could take it from me. What was left for me to do but to follow her lead and write it?

In reading and writing poetry, I no longer needed to think of every bad thing in life, every loss, as being part of God's plan. Rather, I started to see my losses as things that could be named, honored, and, through art, brought into the present, transformed. My poetry obsession had fully taken root, and I started eating all my meals to go so that I could sit alone in the library basement writing poems.

* * *

God speaks directly to the prophet Jeremiah and tells him that he is chosen to serve the Lord. Jeremiah responds by telling God that he does not know how to speak and lists off his inadequacies. His point is clear: God is making a big mistake in choosing him. Despite this resistance, God responds by touching Jeremiah's mouth and appointing him over nations and kingdoms. God calls Jeremiah to warn Judah that they will be sent into captivity by Babylon, but the people fail to listen to him. His family even turns against Jeremiah and plots to kill him. Jeremiah follows the calling of God and speaks for him, but this comes at a price. He becomes a laughingstock and is widely mocked. He is whipped, attacked by a mob, threatened by a king, and accused of treason. Filled with sorrow, Jeremiah questions why God called him to deliver bad news to others. Many scholars refer to him as the "Weeping Prophet." He does not doubt the existence of God, but he questions why he must experience such pain in following him. He knows he can't stay quiet; the words keep pouring forth from his mouth.

I've never felt like a prophet called by God to deliver news to my people. But ever since my days at Hope, I've felt called to write. I didn't know exactly what I had to say or whether anyone would ever read my words. But, since those days in Dr. Glidsan's class, I've known that writing was a calling that I could not shake.

* * *

At the beginning of the semester, Dr. Glidsan broke the class into small writing groups that were supposed to meet weekly.

These meetings accounted for most of my social interaction in college. One of my groupmates, Frank, suggested in an email to the group that we should all meet at Good Time Donuts, a place that I had never heard of. When I arrived there for the first time, I noticed the store's name written in neon block letters. When I walked inside, the only light came from the pastry case and oversize fish tank, and I could tell the store's heat was off. Frank waved at me from the back booth; every other table was empty. He rubbed his hands together and put on a gray hat. When I walked up to the pastry case, I noticed how none of the donut flavors were labeled. Frank could tell that I was overwhelmed and pointed to three of his favorites: a glazed bear claw filled with raspberry, a glazed cruller, and a cream-filled donut covered in chocolate glaze. I ordered all of them. As we walked back to the table, I took a bite of the cruller, which was still warm, and closed my eyes, saying, "This is the best donut that I've ever had in my life." Frank laughed.

"I told you," he said. "They are the best."

My group began meeting every week at the donut shop, and it became my favorite place to write. I noticed over time how the owner was often in the back room wearing a T-shirt and boxers while cutting dough.

I learned through my sessions that Frank led worship at the weekly chapel gatherings at Hope. He often commented about how he never saw me there, and I felt too embarrassed to admit that I'd never attended. He wore oversize glasses and thick shirts bought from local thrift stores, the type of thing worn by everyone you saw hanging out in the coffee shops around town. Throughout the semester, Frank prepared to propose to his girlfriend while wrestling through remnants of his past. He refrained from showing judgment whenever I shared poems about my own experiences with the church.

Our other groupmate, Nicole, spent her free time training as an runner and cheerleader. Her poems mainly expressed regrets over late-night parties. Whenever I read her poems, I felt like I wanted to be invited to these parties, even though, because of my medications, I'd decided to avoid drinking. Her life represented what I wished my college experience looked like. She always arrived at our group meetings after a run, her bleach-blond hair wet from perspiration.

The three of us sat in a dimly lit corner with our notebooks each week. I did not know what a healthy church looked like back then, but I imagined it to be something like my group. None of us shared friends or similar interests. But we connected over our desire to understand and accept suffering.

While I lived in Michigan, this group became the closest thing that I had to a community. Together, we asked God questions. How can we learn to recover from what seems unrecoverable? How do we live with life-altering events, such as receiving a severe mental health diagnosis? How do we keep going when hope seems lost? We never found definite answers, but that didn't stop us from exploring the questions in our poems. God never shouted from the sky to let me know that he was present with me in Michigan, but I can see now that I always had the people I needed to help me move forward.

Halfway through the semester, in March, snow continued to cover the campus despite spring's near arrival. After our group meeting one night, Nicole left to attend a party with friends while Frank and I stayed behind. I finished packing up my notebooks into my purse while Frank sat in the booth across from me. After a long pause, he asked, "Are you still hungry?"

Recalling that I'd missed dinner earlier in the evening, I agreed to get more food, and he got up from the booth, saying, "Come on, I know a place that I think you'd like." We walked down sidewalks coated in ice, passing by the residential homes where students and faculty lived, the humming sound of electric heaters filling the air. Frank combed his fingers through his locks of brown hair, which looked much darker in the night. I studied the freckles dotted around his nose that appeared underneath the streetlights. He pointed at a convenience store on a corner next to a fraternity house. "This place has the best nachos that you'll ever eat," he said. He could tell by my expression that I did not believe him. "I promise," he said.

A bell rang as we walked inside. Right away, I became overwhelmed by what I saw in front of me. Different colored wigs lined the walls. Tacky costume jewelry was placed on several displays in between beer cans and packaged snacks. I watched as college boys stood in the back debating the relative merits of different brands of beer. Frank followed behind me as I took notes in my journal.

"I told you that you'd like it here," he said. I scribbled down everything that I saw: the neon-colored hair extensions, the bottles of cheap perfume, the college boys. I wanted to shape this entire night into a poem. Being there with Frank, I finally felt like I had made a friend.

Frank walked up to the front counter and ordered us a plate of nachos to share. The clerk opened a container of nacho cheese and poured the yellow sauce on top of a bed of chips. I opened the door after Frank paid, surprised by a gust of wind that made me look down toward the sidewalk.

"Here," he said, handing me a chip covered in cheese. I bit into it, struck by the rich cheddar flavor.

"Okay, fine," I said. "You're right. These are pretty good." We began walking down one of the streets lined with homes.

He looked over to me and said, "Are you still a Christian?"

I sensed hesitation in his words, and I could tell he was nervous about asking this question. To delay answering, I kept stuffing chips into my mouth. He tried to explain. "I can never tell from your poems," he said. "You seem to be wrestling with a lot." I could see his breath in the cold air, and my body shivered under my thin wool coat. He took a sweatshirt out of his backpack and handed it to me. I averted my gaze, hoping to avoid making eye contact.

I wasn't sure what to tell Frank. My beliefs would have been unrecognizable to me just a few years earlier, a fact that troubled me. I felt shame at the idea that my faith wasn't obvious. This, to me, was the ultimate sign that I was a bad Christian. But I also felt safe with Frank, the way you feel safe with a friend you've known for years. I felt so safe that I wanted to tell him about all the ways that I felt I'd failed. I wanted to tell him about how I feared my diagnosis was the result of a lack of trust in God. I wanted to tell him about my suicidal ideation. I wanted to tell him how I cared more about Hunter than I cared about God. I wanted to tell him that I'd selfishly harmed my friends by burdening them with my troubles. I wanted to tell him how I'd let my parents down. I wanted to tell him about this one night in Winston-Salem when I got drunk—a grievous sin in my community—and told my friends that I wanted to kill myself.

But I didn't tell him all that. What I did tell him was that I was still trying to figure out where I fit within Christianity.

He paused for a moment, taking in what I'd said. "Well, Jesus always loved the misfits," he said. "Why don't you come to my church sometime?" I told him that I would and kept eating nachos.

When I did attend Frank's church, though, I found it uncomfortably reminiscent of the churches of my youth—strobe lights, drums and electric guitars, guys in skinny jeans and flannel, biceps with Bible verses tattooed on them. I stayed for one song before escaping back to my car.

In the car, I took solace in my own private church, the one I found in poetry. I took out my journal and started writing a sonnet about what I'd just witnessed. It was an admittedly bad poem—including lines comparing myself to an Israelite in the desert and proclaiming, "I am damned"—but it was also a reminder that I could try, however imperfectly, to put my beliefs and feelings into words.

I knew that Dr. Glidsan would have a lot of feedback for me, but that was okay. I was learning how to write the truth, which felt like a form of redemption. Before Dr. Glidsan's class, my daily journal entries were filled with praise to God. But poetry gave me the freedom to question, to doubt, to lament—to engage with God as the person I was, not as the person I thought I had to be. The more I wrote, the more honest my poems became. Each poem was a plea to God to make himself known to me in a new way. It took me years to realize that writing was my preferred way of praying.

* * *

Near the end of the semester, and hoping to find new material for my poems, I accompanied a friend to a nearby tattoo parlor, where she planned to get a new tattoo. We walked in, and I took a seat next to her before immediately opening up my poetry journal. I made a bullet point list of every detail I noticed. The statue of Jesus next to the door. The baby doll's head placed atop a stack of Civil War history books. Photos of clowns alongside renderings of Buddha and Mary, the mother of Christ. Eventually my friend was guided through a pair of saloon doors into a room where she lay down on a table. Above the table I saw the heads of two large animals, a boar and a deer. I then watched as the tattoo artist carefully, methodically dipped his pen in black ink and applied it to my friend's back, drawing the outlines of letters and then filling them in one by one. When he was finished, I could see that the message on my friend's back read: "It's always darkest before the dawn." This was one of my favorite lyrics by Florence and the Machine, and an apt message for my own life. I kept writing down everything I saw.

After my friend dropped me off on campus, I went to the library basement and began writing a poem about the tattoo parlor. The first line read: "We were greeted by zombie portraits and deer heads." I didn't get up from my seat until the poem was finished. Later, looking over my work, I was surprised to find that I'd written something that I liked. It captured all the little details, and it had a sense of humor about them. I titled it "I Lasted Ten Minutes in a Tattoo Parlor," and, at the next class, I turned it in to Dr. Glidsan.

Slowly, and largely below the level of consciousness, poetry was changing the way I interacted with the world. Gone were the days that I walked around campus with my headphones on and my head down. I no longer tried to fill my every moment with some distraction. I was no longer trying to hide. Poetry slowed my mind enough that I could perceive a world outside of my own ruminations. The poet Mary Oliver wrote:

> *Let me*
> *keep my mind on what matters,*
> *which is my work,*
> *which is mostly standing still and learning to be*
> *astonished.*

For me, learning to be astonished meant getting quiet enough to see what was, and had always been, right in front of me. I wrote it all down in my poems—the busy airport, the gas station merchandise, the donut shop, the differences between red and white oak trees. And, if I could learn to see the world around me with such love and reverence, how much more did God love and revere the creation? In my moments of greatest clarity, I knew that God was present in the here and now, and that my belief in him had nothing to do with the changing weather of my emotions. God was there no matter how I felt, and my job was to believe in the little resurrections happening all around me.

In the Gospels, after Christ is crucified and has died on the cross, the curtain of the holy temple is suddenly torn in half. Christ's death, in other words, has made a personal relationship with God available to all. You don't need to be a high priest, or a pastor, or even an especially spiritual person to know God; you can be exactly the person you are. That was what poetry showed me.

During the next poetry class, Dr. Glidsan handed out the latest packet of student poems. Flipping through a few pages, I saw it: my tattoo parlor poem had been chosen.

My classmates were thrilled. Frank even asked if he could read it aloud; I agreed, and he did. After class, Dr. Glidsan pulled me aside and said, "Be proud of yourself. You're really starting to get it."

*　*　*

During our last class of the semester, each student handed out chapbooks of poems that we had written. Mine was entitled *First in Flight*, a reference to North Carolina's state motto. My copies of these chapbooks remain in a box next to my bed.

Sitting together in our usual seats, we offered reflections about what the class had meant to us. It felt like I was in church, hearing people share their faith testimonies.

But it was more than a feeling. This *was* my church, and these were my friends. They were speaking about poetry, and it felt no different from speaking about God. I was so grateful that I could hardly speak, for fear that I'd start crying. We set a self-timer on Dr. Glidsan's phone, and we stood together, posing for a photograph. We wrapped our arms around one another and smiled, and then we left the classroom together. I looked back at the dark room, now empty, knowing without a doubt that this last class with my chosen family would stick with me.

Chapter 7

At the beginning of the summer of 2013, I went with my best friend from high school, Jane, to Walmart. We went there with a specific purpose in mind: to purchase a garden gnome.

With the gnome procured, we got in Jane's car and rode over to David's house. We parked outside and waited. David was eight years my senior, and I knew him from the church I'd attended in high school. Now I saw him as a tall youth leader with light brown eyes. He stood out in a crowd, a result of his funny T-shirts and a laugh that echoed through the church lobby after services. I loved his gap-toothed smile and his taste in music, and I loved the fact that he was the only person in my life who laughed at my dark jokes.

Jane ran up to his front porch and left the gnome on a lawn chair while I kept watch to make sure neighbors didn't see us. The streets remained empty as we drove away. When I got home, I posted photos on Facebook and Instagram with the caption: "Missing Gnome. Offering a baked pie reward." This was my idea of flirtation.

David wasn't the most observant person. Three days went by, and he still hadn't noticed the gnome. Nor, apparently, had he seen my hilarious post. On that third day, David's roommate, returning home late from work, spotted it. But at first he wasn't sure what he saw; the sight of this mysterious shadowy figure caused him to scream, believing he was about to be robbed. He jumped back from the door and was prepared to defend himself against this attacker, only to find the little garden gnome smiling up at him and holding a yellow flower. He brought the gnome inside, assuming David had played a joke on him.

After seeing my social media posts and putting the pieces together, David contacted me via text.

"I'd like a strawberry rhubarb pie in exchange for Chester's ransom," he wrote.

"Deal," I replied.

We planned to meet up after I returned from vacation. Meanwhile, he posted a series of photographs of the gnome all around town. He posted a photo of the gnome in a pastry case at Starbucks with a caption scolding him for breaking health code violations. He posted another of him sitting on a ledge above an interstate bridge, appearing as if he were preparing to take his own life. This, it turned out, was David's own way of flirting with me.

At the time, I had no idea if he considered our looming hangout to be a date, though I certainly did. When I lived in Raleigh, he had reached out to see if I wanted to attend an Andrew Bird concert with him. I turned him down because the idea of live music while depressed seemed like a bad idea. I also wanted to stay very far away from men. Still, for some reason, David and I had stayed in touch over the years.

The morning of our potential date, I researched rhubarb

pie recipes. Before David's text, I hadn't known such a plant existed. I took a bite of one in the grocery store parking lot and immediately spit it out, unsettled by its bitter taste.

When David arrived at the coffee shop later that afternoon, he saw me sitting alone on the front porch and sat in the chair across from me. He took off his sunglasses as he sat down. He wore a Mozart T-shirt and shorts that he created by cutting a pair of old dark jeans with craft scissors. I was drawn to these quirks, to all his little quirks; he wasn't like anyone I'd ever gone out with before. The black metal chair was uncomfortable no matter how I tried to reposition my body. I handed him the strawberry rhubarb pie, and he gave me my garden gnome, which I placed on our table, where he kept watch over our whole discussion.

David walked into the coffee shop and grabbed a fork before coming back to take a bite of pie. "This is better than my grandma's pies," he said. He strategically picked a piece of the rhubarb-and-strawberry slice with his fork. "Is this crust homemade?"

"Yes," I said, lying to him. It was really a frozen Pillsbury crust that I had purchased from the grocery store. I wanted him to think I was a cool professional baker rather than a mediocre aspiring poet. I watched as his brown beard became covered in pie, a fact he failed to notice because he was so focused on taking more and more bites of the pie. I found this endearing.

He crossed his legs, and I noticed the tattoo on his calf depicting a swallow carrying a coconut.

"It's from my favorite Monty Python movie," he said.

"Have you seen *The Holy Grail*?" He placed the Saran wrap back on the pie after finishing about a third of it. I told him that my dad had shown me clips of the film when I was younger, but I never understood the humor. I wasn't used to dates where guys asked me questions.

"Where's your family from?" I asked.

"Nebraska. I followed my parents to the South when my dad got a new job. My relatives were German farmers who settled in a rural town that always smells like beets."

Hearing "Nebraska," I thought of the band Bright Eyes, since they're from there, and I thought of Elliott Smith, who was also from there, along with Bruce Springsteen's *Nebraska* album, with its title track about a serial killer. I thought of large, open cornfields and car rides where you can see clearly for miles. My mind raced. Which of these free associations should I mention? Which topic would demonstrate to David that I was an attentive listener, a deep thinker, and generally a joy to be around? I zeroed in on his mention of German farmers.

"You know," I said, "my great-grandparents survived the Armenian genocide. That genocide served as inspiration for Hitler. And the United States still hasn't acknowledged that what happened to the Armenians was a genocide. Did you know that?"

He shook his head.

"My grandma," I continued, "still holds a grudge against Obama because he promised that he'd formally recognize the genocide. He still hasn't. Can you believe that?"

He shook his head again. He listened as I described the

atrocity, my voice brimming with anger, my words blurring together in one run-on sentence after another, pausing only to take sips of my cold brew coffee. When I finally stopped talking, David took out his phone and showed me some photos from his recent trip to Swaziland. "If you could go anywhere in the world," he asked, "where would you choose?"

I replied instantly: "A concentration camp."

"Oh," he said. "Me too."

Before leaving, David stood up from his chair and said, "I think that we should do this again sometime." I nodded, stunned.

David texted me a few days later that he wanted to take me to dinner but left it to me to choose the restaurant. I immediately picked Waffle House. He said, "Excellent choice," leaving out the fact that he was not a fan of the restaurant or anywhere that might have a questionable health grade. He found the place to be dirty and the food to be too greasy, but he did not want to hurt my feelings. I would come to learn that David is obsessed with cleanliness in a way that I am not.

I wasn't sure if he wanted to meet as friends or if we were going on a date. Meanwhile, my friends and family were shocked that I was even interested in David. Most of them thought after my last breakup and years of being single that I'd sworn off dating altogether. One evening after David finished work, we arrived at the restaurant. I led us to the back booth where I normally sat. David took out a Lysol wipe and began cleaning the table. He picked up his silverware and held it up to the light to make sure that it was clean.

I leaned my body against the window and sat in the booth

as though I were lounging on a couch. Music from the juke-box, selected by teens who apparently wanted to listen to Aaron Carter and Beyoncé, filled the restaurant. I studied the faces of customers sitting alone at the counter with mugs of coffee. I watched from behind the counter as employees mixed chopped hash browns with a combination of cheese, onions, ham, tomatoes, mushrooms, and jalapeño peppers. I discovered while going to college in Winston that you could get Wi-Fi from the Starbucks next door, and I used to go late at night to the restaurant to write term papers while taking bites of my hash browns covered with cheese.

Our waitress came over to deliver the Diet Cokes that we ordered. David had asked to have his without ice, but the waitress had forgotten, and David didn't bother to comment. I ordered a double order of chocolate chip waffles, and David looked up from the menu at our waitress and said, "Can I just have a salad?" I wondered whether this was a red flag. Had I gotten him all wrong?

I tried to appear graceful, eating my waffles carefully with a fork and knife. Had I been there alone, I would've picked them up with my hands. David asked, "Where did you go to high school in Winston? I'm a youth leader and know most of the schools."

"I went to the Southern Baptist one on Peace Haven Road," I replied. "It's something that I'm still recovering from."

He laughed and said, "It's okay, I did Christian home-schooling from kindergarten until twelfth grade."

I had never met anyone who homeschooled for their entire schooling career. We began comparing notes about growing up in Christian education. We both knew more about creationism than evolution. We both knew Christian pop culture references from shows like *McGee and Me!*, *Adventures in Odyssey*, and *VeggieTales*. We both knew all about the Christian film production companies that made knockoffs of secular films. David grew up listening to bands I knew well, like DC Talk and Switchfoot, as well as Christian boy bands like Plus One, who modeled themselves on the Backstreet Boys. We were speaking the same language, and I felt comfortable enough to tell him about the time I faked being filled with the Holy Spirit during middle school youth group.

"Like you actually fell down and pretended?" he asked, laughing.

"Yeah, it all worked until I fell asleep on the floor during worship."

"You know, maybe you have a future in acting."

"That might be more lucrative than a career in writing."

As the stories left my mouth, I realized that I was sharing parts of my life that caused me shame. I asked him questions about his daily life because his calmness and stability fascinated me. Even the relaxed, nonchalant way he leaned back on his side of the booth felt so foreign to who I was. He managed to sit still throughout our dinner while I shifted constantly in my seat.

He scraped his bowl of soggy lettuce covered in ranch dressing and explained, "I'm asleep each night by ten p.m. and awake at five a.m. to run my four-mile route." I hadn't met anyone in my life with so much structure. Despite the fact that every psychiatrist I'd ever had told me that routine was essential for me, I typically failed to follow any clear schedule for more than a few days at a time.

Before leaving, we agreed to keep spending time together. I drove home listening to a playlist of upbeat music including artists like Modest Mouse, Local Natives, and Grizzly Bear for the first time in months. It scared me how much I liked being with David, how easy it felt to be myself with him. But my fear wasn't enough to keep me away from him.

Before I saw David next, I found myself grappling with questions about what a relationship with him might look like. We were both coming out of an evangelical context, which, when it came to dating, meant a few things. It meant that we would certainly not be having sex before marriage. It also meant that the possibility of marriage—and all that marriage entailed—had to be on the table. And what would a married life with David look like? When I was a kid, I read Christian dating books with titles like *I Kissed Dating Goodbye* and *When God Writes Your Love Story*, and I learned that the man I married would be the "spiritual leader" of our relationship. In other words, my future husband would make decisions for us, leading us on a path of holiness. What any of that would ever look like in practice, I didn't know. Was this how David envisioned his future marriage? These were some of the questions and concerns I fretted and obsessed over between dates.

But then there was also the problem of my diagnosis. I hadn't told him about it. And ever since my diagnosis, I'd always suspected, deep down, that I wasn't stable enough to be married. I believed I needed to heal before I could have a partnership with anybody. But would I ever be healed enough?

One month after our first date, David and I had a talk in a department store. I was soon to return to Michigan for school, and I wondered if he wanted to continue our relationship. We were standing in line together so David could buy a pair of pants, and James Blunt's "You're Beautiful"—the most annoying song ever composed—was playing in the background.

"I want you to be my girlfriend," he said.

I nodded without speaking, nervous about what I was going to say and making a mental note of the fact that James Blunt provided the soundtrack for our first moment in an official relationship. Still, even with my fears, I knew that this is what I wanted, and it felt almost too good to be true.

We stood in the store entrance for a few moments as families walked past us. He gave me a hug, and we went our separate ways.

Our first fight as a couple happened mere days later, over dinner at an Italian restaurant where waiters sang opera songs while people ate. Before arriving, I'd decided that I was going to tell David about my bipolar diagnosis.

But I soon realized that this would not be the night I shared that information. While telling me about one of his college classes, in which he'd learned about suicide prevention campaigns, he said, "Sometimes I feel like people attempt suicide for attention, not because they actually want to die."

I got up from my chair, shaking with rage. "You're wrong," I said. "You don't know what you're talking about." I raced to the bathroom. There it was, the confirmation I needed. I'd tell him about my diagnosis and he'd think of me as an attention-seeker. I was too much for him, and I was unlovable in general. He was sure to cast me out of his life and never look back.

Emerging from the bathroom, I looked over at the entrance, eyeing the couples holding electronic buzzers as they awaited an empty booth, and I assessed my options. I could make a run for it; the door was right there. Sure, David would never talk to me again, but that was okay. He'd be better off. And I didn't need him anyway, what with his ignorant opinions about mental illness. Yes, running was a good idea.

But as I looked at David alone at the table, taking tiny bites of bread dipped in olive oil, I knew I couldn't leave him. I sat down, and he apologized immediately.

"I'm guessing you disagree with me," he continued. "Do you want to tell me why?"

For a moment, I considered telling him my story, but instead I answered with a general observation about how suicidal ideation was more complex than he claimed, and often people who attempted suicide were living with a sense of desperation that was hard for most people to fathom. That I myself knew this desperation well would have to be a story for another dinner. But, by the way he looked at me, I sensed that he knew exactly what I was talking about and *who* I was talking about.

"You're right," he said. "I was being too simplistic, and I'm sorry."

Later, it occurred to me that my outburst at dinner was the first time I'd vocally disagreed with a man I was dating. This would have been unthinkable just a few years before, so thoroughly was I convinced that a good Christian man wanted a meek, submissive partner. But David was flipping those notions upside down, and I was discovering, to my surprise, that I might be lovable exactly as I was. Just maybe.

A few weeks later, I met with Whitney to talk about my new relationship. I sprawled on her couch, holding a pillow over my face.

"I feel kind of sick," I explained. "Nauseated. Because of how happy I am with him. Is my body incapable of tolerating happiness? Is this how happy people feel?"

The stakes felt very high for me. My previous relationship had ended in a breakup, and that breakup, along with its subsequent fallout (being asked to leave my church after being called a "spiritual stumbling block" by my pastor, experiencing debilitating depression, and so on), had destroyed me. I couldn't go through that again.

Whitney looked at her clock and informed me that we had only ten minutes left. I decided to ask her what I really wanted to know: "How do I know that my bipolar diagnosis won't make him leave?"

"You can't *know* the answer to that, Anna," she said. "But these things aren't about *knowing*. Life's not about *knowing*. Sometimes, we must be willing to take a leap of faith."

* * *

The author of the book of Exodus refers to Noah as "righteous" who "walked faithfully with God," standing in stark contrast to the wicked and evil world around him.

Whenever I read this as a child, I wondered why God considered the world to be so evil. Maybe people back then were murdering one another and stealing from malls, I reasoned. Fed up with all the wickedness, God decides to destroy the world but to spare Noah, his family, and two of each kind of animal. He tells Noah to build an ark, even providing precise measurements and a basic floor plan.

Thunderstorms during my childhood were always a cause for concern. I had nightmares, worried that God was destroying the world. As an adult, I found myself less interested in God's rationale for destroying the world and more interested in the absurd, almost comic predicament Noah finds himself in. He builds that ark for *years*. Surely people walk by and laugh, thinking him foolish, untethered to reality. But he keeps building, abandoning himself utterly to God's will. He builds because he trusts.

As my relationship with David deepened, I wondered how it looked from the outside. Though no one said so, I suspected that some of my friends thought it was doomed from the start. If they had said it, I wouldn't have blamed them. I didn't have a great track record of stability, of seeing things through. No matter how it looked, though, I felt in a way I couldn't explain that I was doing what God intended for me to do: building a life with David. God hadn't given me any measurements, and the ark David and I were building lacked a clear floor plan, but I knew we needed to build it, and that it would carry us through whatever storms were still to come.

* * *

Before I left for school, David drove to my parents' house to say goodbye to me. He leaned against his old Buick with his hands in his pockets as I approached him in the driveway. Up until that point, he had tried kissing me on multiple occasions, but I shyly responded by turning away or looking at the ground. When I saw him this time, I walked over to him before he could even say anything and grabbed the sides of his face and pulled him toward me. As we kissed, I felt him put his arms around me. I did not want to run away. I wanted to stay frozen in that moment with him.

When David got home, his roommate saw him walk in with a smile on his face and said, "She must have finally kissed you."

* * *

Back at school, I was grappling with the fact that I still hadn't told David about my diagnosis. On some level, it felt unfair, as though I wasn't letting him know exactly what he was getting himself into. After days of ignoring his texts, too afraid to have a conversation, I asked him if we could talk over video chat.

"You know when I left that gnome on your porch?" I said. "That's not something I normally do. I was having a manic episode. I have bipolar disorder."

With that, the words started pouring out of me. I listed symptoms. I described the chaos of which I was capable. I presented what I understood to be the cold reality: people with bipolar disorder tend to make difficult partners in romantic relationships. Anyone who ended up with me would have to weather a fair degree of turbulence, and there was simply no getting around that. All while I talked, David looked ahead at his screen, without raising his eyebrows or appearing surprised.

When I finally finished speaking, David sat quietly for a moment. Then he said, "Anna, we all have our personal demons. I have some, too." He proceeded to list what he understood to be his many shortcomings and sins, including the time he tried to burn down his parents' house.

This was my kind of guy. We dated through the school year, and when I was home on break, we spent every day together. He was the first person I'd ever dated who would simply be with me through my mental health episodes. There were nights when I'd ask him to stay on the phone with me, and he would. There were days when I felt like I was spiraling out of control again—a constant fear for me—and he'd gently return me to reality, with patience and humor. Once, after my psychiatrist switched my meds, having me take something called Latuda, David had flowers delivered to my dorm with a note: "Congrats on the Latuda!" I, meanwhile, was teaching David to name his own emotions. I knew a lot about feelings, and David knew a lot about calmly moving through situations.

Over the summer, I got an internship at a poetry press, and I kept spending all my time with David. On the night before I was set to return to school, we watched a movie called *Troll*, a poorly written film about trolls taking over an apartment complex. At the film's conclusion, I got up from the couch and started pacing.

"Where do you see this relationship going?" I demanded.

"Anna?" he replied.

Suddenly gripped by the need to *know* and by a fear that everything could be taken from me suddenly and without warning, I asked him again. Where did he see our relationship going?

He sat back with his hands behind his head and responded with a matter-of-factness one might adopt while describing that day's weather. "I wouldn't be with you if I didn't want to marry you," he said.

"Oh," I said, plopping back down on the couch next to him. "How do you know that?"

"I just know," he said.

Later he'd tell me about the precise moment he knew, a moment he'd described to his sister just hours after it happened. It was at the Waffle House, when I told him a story about how my childhood dog, a pug named Moses, got so scared of our vacuum cleaner that his eyes actually bulged out of his head and dangled from their sockets. (My mom popped them back in.)

There on the couch, I rested my head against his shoulder, imagining our marriage. And then it occurred to me: I was *imagining our marriage*, which meant that this person saw me in their future, a future that may very well stretch across many years. And what would those years include? I pictured myself playing in the yard with our child as David came home from work. It was almost inconceivable to me; I'd spent so much of my life feeling like getting through a single day was hard enough.

We started discussing how this would all work. I told him that I needed to go to graduate school for writing. He told me he'd be willing to take a consulting job so that I could go to school wherever I wanted.

The next morning, my mom drove me to the airport. "How did last night with David go?" she asked.

"I think I'm going to marry him."

Chapter 8

Forty-five minutes before I was set to marry David, I managed to lose my heels. Months earlier, I had spent two hundred dollars on this pair of metallic heels, the most I'd ever spent on a pair of shoes. They sat in a white shoebox wrapped in tissue paper on the top shelf of my closet up until our wedding day: April 12, 2015.

My bridesmaids and I searched through each of our bags in the back room of the wedding venue. My best friend, Jane—my coconspirator in the garden gnome incident—took charge and called the Airbnb where we had stayed the night prior.

She sighed as she hung up the phone. "She hasn't seen them," she said.

I sat down on the couch and pulled a pillow over my face. "I just wanted this day to go perfectly." We each looked at one another, unsure of where else to search. One of my bridesmaids, Abby, started to cry. "This is all my fault!" she said. "It was my job to bring everything!"

Her eye makeup began to smear as she continued to cry. My five bridesmaids began speaking back and forth while I threw everything out from each of our bags, hoping to find the shoes. They watched as I turned the room into a disaster area. I'd planned to keep those shoes in my closet for years to come, a sentimental reminder of what was supposed to be the most memorable day of my life. And now they were gone. My wedding planner appeared in the doorway and asked, "Are you sure you've looked everywhere?" I told her about all the places that we'd checked.

I sat on the ground in defeat. Casey, my friend since kindergarten, crossed her arms and began developing a plan. She tucked strands of her blond hair behind her ears the way she always did when concentrating. Casey always acted rationally in emergency situations, which was exactly why we were friends. "Let me text my mom," she said. "She can buy you some on her way to the venue."

Jane tried to calm me down by switching my mind to something else. "At least you'll get to have sex soon!" she said. Everyone laughed, except for me.

"I don't need another thing to stress me out right now," I snapped. I briefly thought about David seeing me naked for the first time. I gulped down more coffee to try to calm myself down.

As we waited for the shoes, with twenty minutes to spare, my five bridesmaids placed their hands on my shoulders and prayed for me and my marriage. Of the five bridesmaids, three were friends who'd known me and stuck by me since before my diagnosis. The other two were my older sister and David's younger sister.

My sister led the prayer. "God," she said, "help people see you in how Anna and David love each other."

Upon the prayer's conclusion, I paced around the room, reviewing the flash cards on which I'd written my vows. "I will fail you," they read. "I will disappoint you. But in failures and shortcomings, I won't back out. I won't give up on you or our marriage, regardless of circumstances." In our relationship, in our love, we'd built our ark.

We heard a knock on the door, and in walked Casey's mom, waving a pair of gold flip-flops in the air, which she'd found at a nearby discount store. I ran over and hugged her, slipping on the shoes, which were at least a size too big and adorned with the ugliest rhinestones the world had ever seen. My wedding planner rushed in and shouted, "Ten minutes until showtime!"

As my dad walked me down the aisle, he whispered for me to look up and smile. My eyes glanced over at our guests, all standing from their seats, smiling at me as I passed by. I felt my heart beat faster and faster. But then I saw Blake, a high school friend who went walking late at night with me in Raleigh grocery stores while we were both depressed. I saw Mattie, who lay underneath Christmas lights with me in Winston when life felt unbearable. I saw Lauren and Kara, who stayed up late with me to discuss God night after night. I saw Meredith, who threw toilet paper with me all over a bathroom when another medication was not working. Then there were my bridesmaids, who drove late at night for milkshakes with me, who put up with me driving my car in a ditch, who drove with me for hours without a clear destination, who wrote letters to me at every college I attended, who never complained when I slept through yet another coffee date. I became overwhelmed with a sense of gratitude for those who helped me get to where I was in life.

I looked forward and made eye contact with David, who

was standing at the front of the altar, pacing back and forth in anticipation. He began to laugh to hide the fact that he could not stop crying. Just before my dad and I passed by my family in the front rows, I offered David a wave and he gave me one in return, as if we were the only two in the room. The level of commitment that we were making to each other hit both of us as we stood across from each other. I held his hands and looked into his eyes, dreaming of building a life together.

During his vows, David pulled out a piece of paper from his back pocket and read, "My love isn't perfect, unfortunately. I can't love perfectly like Jesus can."

I found this comforting, his acknowledgment of our human frailty, our inability to do anything—let alone marriage—perfectly. Frailty was something I believed I knew well. But I also knew grace, and I knew how grace was often found, or perhaps exclusively found, amid our shoddy, imperfect little lives, among the fragments we try so hard to gather into a beautiful whole. Grace finds us there. It can even find us when we've lost our shoes, and the ones we're wearing don't fit.

"We will make countless amazing memories with each other," he continued, "but we're also going to face challenges far harder than we've already faced. And still, my deepest desire is to look at you and love you." His tears stained the ink as he read from the page.

Fittingly, the microphones on the stage had accidentally been turned off; no one could hear the promises we made to each other that day but us.

As David continued to read, I noticed that snot was running down his face. Add that to the list: God is with us even when we're covered in snot. His groomsmen huddled together, searching for a Kleenex, finding one, and passing it to David just before it was time to kiss me. My husband grabbed the sides of my face and brought it toward him and kissed me as if we were alone. I heard our friends begin to cheer with his face still pressed against mine. We walked down the aisle and went into an elevator, where we were finally alone for a moment before reaching the reception.

He glided his hand down my back, which made me wonder if our first night together would make me feel closer to him, what it would feel like to have his body against mine, until the doors opened, revealing our friends and family. He reached for my hand and led me out into the cheering crowd.

* * *

Christ's first recorded miracle takes place at a wedding. Jesus, his mother, and his disciples are at a wedding in Galilee when the wine runs out. Jesus notices six stone water jars in the serving area, and he tells his disciples to fill them with water. The guests are delighted to discover that Jesus has turned the water into wine. He is able to take something ordinary and transform it.

At my wedding reception with David, we didn't serve any wine, or any other alcoholic beverages. Instead, we served an endless supply of Diet Coke and coffee, our favorite drinks. As I looked around at my friends, gathered at tables or out on the dance floor, I thought, *If this isn't a miracle, I don't know what it is.* A friend of mine walked up to me as I ate a stack of food and said, "We never thought you'd get married." With my fork I lifted a waffle drenched in maple syrup and smiled. "I know," I said. "Me neither."

* * *

Back at our hotel that night, David and I had sex for the first time.

I suppose such an occasion feels like a big deal for just about everybody. In evangelical culture, it's a big deal as well, but in a different way because of how sex relates to spirituality. For a long time, I believed my sexual desires and lust could result in going straight to hell. The solution to this awful predicament was marriage.

Considering my years of instruction in sexual purity, I thought that my first time might feel awkward. But, with David, it felt utterly natural, a logical extension of the intimacy we'd already developed.

I emerged from the bathroom in a black lace slip that I'd been embarrassed to buy but felt sexy in. David sat on the couch, his hands against his sides, his nervousness not well disguised. Normally I am self-conscious about my body, but I wasn't that night. I reached for him without fear, wanting to be seen by him, known by him.

I took off his pants, making note of his dinosaur-patterned boxers. He reached behind me, pulling down the straps of my slip and sliding off my lace underwear. He held my face and kissed me. Surprised by my own confidence, I climbed on top of him.

When we finished, we lay naked on the bed, and I traced the outline of his spine. I also saw things I'd never noticed before, like the mole on his right shoulder and the way he crinkled his nose. I felt grateful to know that I would have many years to notice even more—all the little details.

But even in my gratitude, I wasn't unencumbered by the past. As I pulled the sheets up to cover my body, I had a suspicion that I'd done something wrong, that maybe I was wrong. Maybe that was to be expected once I acted on desires I'd spent my whole life suppressing, for fear of divine punishment. Even so, I'd experienced enough of life by then to know that these feelings could be endured—that they said far more about the smallness of the world around me than they said about me. I looked over at my husband, wondering what he was thinking.

"Let's go get some steak," he said.

Chapter 9

David and I entered our married lives with our eyes open, knowing full well that it wouldn't be the answer to all of life's problems or the explanation of all of life's mysteries. We expected hardship; we said as much in our vows. But I don't know that we fully understood how challenging it could become.

A big part of marriage, we soon discovered, was learning to live with certain givens. One of those givens was the fact that had followed me since the age of eighteen: I had a mind that routinely attacked me. I had a mental health condition that dramatically reduced my life expectancy and made it harder for me to live anything like a normal life. And so, even though I experienced times of reprieve—writing poems, being with David, reflecting gratefully on the world around me—the time would always come again when my mind would convince me that all was lost, that hope was groundless, that I was doomed.

One of those times, as it turned out, happened on our honeymoon in April 2015. I ate too much Nutella gelato and started manically researching bipolar divorce statistics, looking for confirmation of what I felt I already knew deep down: David would leave me someday. But he put his hand on my shoulder and said, "We will beat the statistics. Loving you means loving your missing brain chemicals, too."

Another one of those times was when I returned home from our honeymoon and collapsed into another depressive episode. David, as promised, had taken a consulting job in Boston, the point of which was to enable me to go to whatever graduate school I wanted. He traveled to Boston every other week while I stayed at our home in Winston-Salem. We put his house in Winston up for sale, in preparation for a move to Washington, DC, where I received a full ride to study writing. But after the house was sold in May, I confessed doubts about being mentally and emotionally equipped to enroll. Voicing my fears led to me scheduling a psychiatric appointment in Boston for June. My parents paid for me to fly up with David and meet with one of the best doctors in the country. That hour-long session left me with an even deeper sense of hopelessness when I was diagnosed with what's known as "treatment-resistant bipolar depression." That's exactly what it sounds like: my depression resists treatment. A new medication might work for a few months, but inevitably a time will arrive when it ceases to be effective and I'm sent back to square one. The psychiatrist put me on lithium and told me that graduate school should wait. He also told David that he'd have to have a more active role in taking care of me, which meant a job in Boston was out of the question.

For years, I'd understood lithium to be a last resort for treating bipolar disorder, one whose side effects could be severe. Lithium was supposed to be used for only the most serious cases—and now that I was being put on lithium, I had to accept that I was one of those cases. The psychiatrist told me that I'd have to get my blood tested every week to ensure that

I was getting a proper dosage and explained the risks involved in lithium toxicity: blurred vision, nausea, tremors, vomiting, brain fog, memory loss. Sensing my apprehension, he added that lithium was hugely popular in the 1920s for its healing properties, even being added to soda. (The fact that cocaine had also been used in Coca-Cola products didn't occur to me at the time.)

So, there we were, newly married, and all our plans, our whole vision for our married life, lay in tatters. And I couldn't help but feel like it was my fault.

* * *

For Christians, regardless of denomination, the death and resurrection of Christ is the central claim of the faith, the foundation upon which everything else rests. St. Paul writes in the book of Corinthians: "And if Christ has not been raised, our preaching is useless and so is your faith." The Gospels all agree about the basic contours of the story. After being accused by the religious and political authorities of his day, Jesus is nailed to a cross, a form of punishment intended to convey to onlookers the utter worthlessness of the victim. He hangs there for several hours and eventually dies. Christians commemorate the day of Christ's death each year on Good Friday.

Jesus is taken down from the cross, his body is wrapped in cloth, and he is placed in a tomb before a large stone covers its entrance. On the third day, a Sunday, two of his followers—two women—go to visit the tomb. As they approach, they ask themselves how they'll ever be able to roll that stone away. But when they get there, they find that the stone has already been removed. An angel greets them inside the tomb, saying, "Why do you look for the living among the dead? He is not here; but he has risen!" This is the occasion Christians celebrate on Easter, the day of Christ's victory over death.

Ever since I was a little kid, though, I wondered about the day between Good Friday and Easter Sunday, the day the Lord was stuck in a tomb. For Jesus's friends and disciples—the people who loved him—that Saturday must have been desolate. They had believed in him; they had placed their hope in him; their dream of a new world relied entirely on him. And that dream was dead.

* * *

I was right to worry about lithium. The brain fog was severe. I tried to throw David a thirtieth birthday party in August and ended up forgetting how to shop for food. Four separate trips to the store resulted in my still having only one pound of ground beef for a party of twenty. I'd also forgotten about half the ingredients necessary to make him his favorite kind of pie. He ended up ordering his own food for the party and thanked me very much for the thought, which was what counted. Not long after, I passed out on a neighbor's lawn while jogging. Instead of getting off lithium, I decided to throw away my running shoes.

David took a job at Duke Hospital in Durham, North Carolina, and we bought a house there. I started seeing a new psychiatrist, this one named Dr. Paktar. The first thing I noticed when I walked into his office were the framed photos of his two children on various family vacations, as well as his collection of medicine bottles on his bookcase. Rows of framed awards lined an entire wall. I was also struck by his gentle, kind demeanor. The first thing he said to me was: "What matters to you?"

I replied by telling him that I wanted to be a stable partner to David but wasn't sure that I could be. I also told him about how I'd quit running because of lithium.

"Well," he said, "it's time to stop that medication. You don't need to sacrifice any more of your life because of this disease."

I proceeded to tell him about my dream of writing a book someday, how I wanted to go to graduate school to complete a manuscript.

"You can accomplish that," he said. "I have several patients who are successful professors at Duke and who also have bipolar disorder. I've worked with corporate lawyers with bipolar disorder. This disease can be managed. It doesn't have to ruin your life." With those words, Dr. Paktar made a new world visible to me.

*　*　*

Three months after my first meeting with Dr. Paktar, my health began to improve. I began volunteering at a senior center, getting back into a routine. Wellbutrin, the medication that he prescribed, began working. But as my health got better, David revealed that he'd been struggling with his own inner darkness. He couldn't quite locate the reasons for it, but he'd started having the nagging feeling that everyone in his life would be better off if he were dead. He told me this as he sat on the edge of our bed, looking down at the floor.

"When did this start?" I asked.

"I forgot to write the date in my diary," he said. "I really just haven't wanted to put more on your plate. You're already dealing with so much."

I was struck by a range of emotions. I was afraid for my husband. I had an overwhelming desire to try to help him, to fix the situation. And then I had emotions that, in turn, made me feel ashamed for having them. I worried that this was my fault, that maybe I really was bad for this person. I worried that I hadn't noticed that my husband was this depressed. Was it because I was constitutionally self-centered, so preoccupied with having my own mental health needs addressed that I couldn't see when a loved one was in pain? It was certainly true that many of our dinner conversations revolved around my diagnosis.

David went to the bathroom, carrying on with his nightly routine as though nothing had happened. As I lay next to him that night, I felt an urge to hold him or pray aloud for him, but the only words I had for God were angry words, so I stayed silent.

A few days later, we attended a game night and bonfire with the only people we knew in Durham, some folks from a local church group. The group consisted entirely of married couples. Lit tiki torches bordered the white picket fence around the backyard. I watched as couples held each other by the fire with ease as David and I awkwardly stood several feet away from each other. Their stillness made marriage appear almost effortless.

David grabbed a beer from a red cooler, and another guy in the group asked him if he'd watched the Duke football game.

I knew for sure that David did not watch the game, would never have watched the game, and had no interest in hearing about the game. Still, he listened patiently to a play-by-play recap of the fourth quarter and stared into the fire.

A woman from the group pulled me aside, running her fingers through her long brown hair while she spoke. She observed that David and I both looked exhausted. I took a sip of my Diet Coke. "We've been struggling," I said.

She put her arm around me. "Has Christ been at the center of your marriage? Are you praying together?" she asked.

"Do you really think that makes marriage easier?" I replied, trying to keep my feelings of anger at bay.

"Oh, absolutely," she said. Problem solved.

I was used to this way of thinking about faith. Are you having a hard time? You must be doing something wrong. Are you feeling sad? Then you've only got to rely even more on God. It's a perspective that sees faith as a kind of contract with the Almighty. If I do this, God will do this. If I fail, then I will be justly punished.

From time to time, I still lapse into this way of thinking. But in my clearer moments I can see that it's really rooted in a desire for control, a desire to make reality manageable. A desire to make God manageable. We are afraid of what might befall us, so we act like modern-day versions of Job's friends, offering our neatly packaged explanations for why others suffer. It's easy to criticize Job's friends, but I see their actions as deeply human, however flawed they may be.

A few weeks later, Dr. Paktar referred David to a psychiatrist with whom he shared an office. This psychiatrist put

David on an antidepressant called Lexapro that had a dramatic and almost immediate impact. The worst of his depressive thinking ceased. I saw him returning to his old self.

"You know," he said once, "seeing everything you went through made it easier for me to accept help. You normalized it all for me."

* * *

Some theologians, particularly in Catholic and Episcopal communities, describe the death and resurrection of Christ as revealing what's known as the Paschal mystery, a cycle of suffering, death, and transformation that we all experience many times over the course of our lives. There's no resurrection without the cross, some say. This wasn't a concept described in the evangelical churches in which I grew up.

Reading the Gospels, I'm struck by the disciples' reluctance to believe that Jesus has really risen from the dead. Examples abound. You've got one scene where they're all hanging out in Jerusalem, in what's known as the Upper Room, having heard rumors that Christ had returned, and they're still not sure. You've got the scene in the Gospel of John where Mary Magdalene sees Jesus at the tomb but doesn't recognize him. The most famous example of this phenomenon is probably Doubting Thomas, the disciple who refused to believe in the resurrection until he literally stuck his fingers in the risen Christ's wounds. But even in the face of Thomas's doubts, Jesus reaches out his own hands without rebuking Thomas. He responds with love. Perhaps even he knows the absurdity of the mystery that we believe in and shape our lives around.

To accept the new life you're being offered, you have to let go of your old life. You have to let go of your illusions. That's what I see Christ's friends and followers trying to do in these stories: let go of what they *thought* Christ was going to do and be, and accept the new life God is offering them.

For me, this doesn't mean that God needs suffering to bring about some better outcome. It does mean, though, that God never abandons us in our suffering. And it means he can bring something good even out of our suffering. But can we accept it?

David and I had begun our married lives with one set of hopes and expectations, and those had to give way to other hopes and expectations. As I watched him grapple with his own mental health and seek support for it, I came to love and appreciate this man in a new and deeper way. Reflecting on childhood spiritual experience, C. S. Lewis had written that he'd been "surprised by joy." I think maybe I was surprised by love—by how deep it can go, by how it accompanies and sustains you even in your darkest hour, when you're walking down a road whose end point you can't see.

* * *

The Gospel of Luke tells a story about two men walking along a road, talking about the death of Christ, when they encounter a stranger. They invite the stranger to walk with them, and they tell him what's happened: a man named Jesus, thought to be the messiah, the one who would change everything, had died the death of a criminal. Rather than accepting their story at face value, the stranger argues with them. He explains how everything happened exactly the way it had to happen. Arriving home, the men invite the stranger inside to eat with them. When the stranger breaks the bread, the men finally realize who he is—the risen Christ himself—and he vanishes as suddenly as he had appeared. I love the way the Gospel writer describes the moment they see him: "Then their eyes were opened and they recognized him."

Their eyes were opened and they recognized him, even on what might have been one of the worst, most traumatic days of their lives.

As we settled into our new lives, David and I made a nighttime ritual of sitting next to each other and coloring in coloring books. David always chose drawings of fish with different patterned scales, swimming among textured coral and seashells. He spent hours on a single picture, making sure that each scale was perfectly shaded. I watched as he moved his pencil in small strokes, meticulously staying within the lines. I remember these nights with great fondness, even nostalgia, because I see that this was when we were learning to simply be present for each other. Just the two of us, walking along the road, or sitting on a couch, with coloring books on our laps.

We were learning to see the healing power of simply being together, in a shared vulnerability. We were learning to accept the good that had been salvaged. In those moments, when our eyes were opened, we were learning to recognize the wounded Lord in the breaking of bread, in the affirming words of doctors, in receiving the right prescriptions, and in sitting beside each other as we tried to stay inside the lines.

Chapter 10

For Durham to really feel like our home, David and I knew we needed to find a church community. Our shared religious traumas made the task challenging; we didn't want to end up at a church that reinforced the same harmful dogmas we were trying to escape.

Since moving to Durham, we had tried to become part of one church community—the one that held backyard cook-outs complete with sports talk and marriage advice—and the results had been less than ideal. David and I had never quite felt that we fit there, and when the assistant pastor told us explicitly that we weren't a good fit for his congregation, our suspicions were confirmed. He told us that we needed a lot more mental health support than his church could provide. So, we left.

During my research, I happened upon Resurrection Church, a nondenominational church that seemed promising. This church wasn't like anything we were used to. Congregants held events about the intersection of theology and the arts. They hosted screenings of spiritual films, including one of my favorites, Martin Scorsese's *Silence*. They supported the local community through initiatives that addressed housing, racial justice, hunger, and services for people leaving prison and jail.

The thing that really sold me on Resurrection, though, was an upcoming lecture series on the book of Lamentations, a book in the Old Testament and one of my favorite books in the whole Bible.

* * *

Scholars are undecided on who wrote Lamentations, but they generally agree that it was written after the destruction of Jerusalem in 586 BCE. The author describes the overwhelming destruction of his homeland: starving children, cannibalism, women being slain with swords. In Hebrew, the word *lament* is *hikya*, which means *how* or *alas!* This book has been a companion to me ever since my diagnosis. When I lived in Michigan, it was the only book of the Bible I read with any regularity. One morning while skipping class, I flipped to a random page, hoping to find a message from God, and landed on Lamentations 3. Verses 2–3 struck me: "He has driven me away and made me walk / in darkness rather than light; / indeed, he has turned his hand against me / again and again, all day long."

But that's not where the story ends. Lamentations 3 opens with this earnest expression of grief, but soon it moves to words of consolation, then to words dripping with a desire for revenge, and then back to words that express confidence in God's faithfulness. It seems to me that so much of what it is to be a human being is captured in these words. They continue to teach me that sorrow, affliction, anger, and hope can all exist within one soul, without canceling out one another.

* * *

A week after finding Resurrection online, David and I attended a service there. The sanctuary that we walked into was nothing impressive to me. The tinted yellow walls appeared like they needed several fresh coats of paint, and the golden chandeliers seemed out of place. About fifteen minutes after the service was supposed to begin, I whispered to David: "Shouldn't the service have started by now?"

From the doorway where he was greeting people as they entered, Pastor Pat overheard me. "We're not the most formal church," he said. "We normally start when people arrive."

* * *

The worship leader that morning was a woman named Katie. She wore dark jeans, and her long blond hair was pulled over to one side. She took the stage with an acoustic guitar strapped across her shoulder. She approached the microphone with her mouth lined with red lipstick and said, "Let's stand and sing together." Behind her there was a large screen on which the lyrics would be projected. "This is one I wrote myself."

I felt my body tense as everyone in the congregation, including David, stood to sing. My tendency to analyze every feeling I had during worship services made it hard for me to sing along with the hymns; I often found myself questioning whether I really meant the words I was singing. I closed my eyes and leaned my head against the wall, listening as Katie's voice filled the room. The words of the song were a plea directly to God, a plea for justice here on earth. She kept playing all throughout the morning—songs about loneliness, about the longing of the human heart, about a God who is present in our pain. These songs were a far cry from the high-energy jams played at the churches of my youth, songs with thrashing drums whose lyrics insisted upon God's awesome power and humanity's sinful nature. Back in those churches, I would raise my hands high and sway and praise God, but I now see that my main motivation was to have others see my devotion to worship and approve. Katie's songs were different; the quality of her voice was different. Or maybe I was different, too, and had been made ready through hard experience to receive this moment of connection. In any event, as Katie kept singing songs like "Heal Us," "Pass Me Not, O Gentle Savior," and "Wounded Healer," I eventually opened my eyes and stood, singing with everyone else.

David and I kept attending Resurrection for the next three weeks, getting to know some of the regulars and feeling genuinely at home in a church community for the first time in years. On that fourth Sunday, Pastor Pat spotted us and asked if we'd like to come over to his home that night for dinner.

When we arrived, Pat greeted us with a big smile. He had on a Tampa Bay Rays ball cap and a T-shirt for one of his favorite local bands, Hiss Golden Messenger. His dining room table was covered with ingredients to make pizza, and he instructed us to pick the toppings we wanted for our own personal pizzas. Pat's beautiful wife, Rachel, walked in wearing a taupe maxi dress, which made me want to immediately ask her where she shopped; somehow, though, I refrained. Two more church members arrived after us, a pair of sisters who had recently moved from Seattle. The younger of the two would end up becoming my best friend in Durham.

As we sat down for dinner, I had to acknowledge to myself that I was having a delightful time with what seemed to be delightful people. But my years of church experience had taught me to maintain a skeptical distance. What was the catch? At any moment, I figured, Pat would start talking about himself, recounting his many spiritually heroic feats and assuring us of the superiority of his particular congregation.

That wasn't what happened. Instead, he asked about us—about what brought us to Durham, about our lives of faith. He asked about what church we attended before Resurrection. David and I glanced at each other, considering whether to tell him about the last church we'd been asked to leave. "The closest I've come to enjoying church," I said, "was when I took a poetry class in college."

"What do you mean by that?" he asked.

I told him all about the class, how it felt like a place where people were engaging with life's mysteries in a spirit of love. I explained that it was in writing poetry that I finally learned how to address God. It turned out that Pat, too, had a mild poetry obsession, and he and I started trading names and titles of our favorite poets and collections.

"That class you took," Pat said, "I think that's what church should be like."

For Pat, the church's agenda in the world should be simple. The church should be a place where diverse human communities can share life together, free from fear and guilt. The church should be a source of hope and healing. It should be a refuge.

On the ride home that night, I burst into tears. David

looked over at me, puzzled. "What's wrong?" he said. "I thought that went well." It had gone well. It was the first time in my life that I felt seen and understood by a pastor. Pastor Pat didn't offer simplistic answers to faith's mysteries. He lived the mysteries alongside us. It's been nearly a decade since I met Pastor Pat, and I know he's exactly the type of Christian St. Paul had in mind when he said, "Rejoice with those who rejoice; mourn with those who mourn." In other words, meet your people where they are and accompany them. That's what Pat does.

The next time I attended a service at Resurrection, Pat announced that Heather, the church's co-pastor, would be delivering the day's sermon. I realized that this meant I'd be hearing a woman preach for the first time in my life.

Heather stood at the podium, adjusted her glasses, and read a verse from Lamentations: "Is it not from the mouth of the Most High that both calamities and good things come?" She looked up from her notes. "Today's sermon," she said, "is going to be my personal testimony, which deals with depression."

I wasn't sure what to expect. Based on past experience, discussions of mental health in church typically led to admonitions about praying away your mental illness, or testimonies to God's miraculous healing power. I rushed to the bathroom to splash some water on my face. As I made my way back to my seat, I heard Heather describing health struggles within her family and the impact they had on her own mental health. "I feel like I can safely tell you," she said, "God is okay with you not being okay. And God would rather you admit it and invite him into it than to try to hang on to it yourself."

She went on to discuss the importance of lamenting our suffering. "Without lament," she said, "there isn't much of a reason for hope. The trick for me, at least, is to keep centering all of this on God and remembering who God is and what he's done." Her testimony didn't involve a solution to her problems, but simply rested on who she believed God was.

After the sermon, David and I decided to attend the post-service potluck, hoping to speak to Heather. I got behind her in line, and I told her I struggled with depression, too. She gave me a hug and offered to get coffee with me sometime.

* * *

My favorite example of a lament in the Bible is not found in the book of Lamentations, but is uttered by Christ himself, in the Garden of Gethsemane on the night before his crucifixion. The scene is depicted in all four Gospels, and it reveals the depths of Christ's sorrow and uncertainty. He knows that he may soon be killed, and he doesn't want that to happen. "My Father," he says, "if it is possible, may this cup be taken from me."

He's in so much anguish that his body begins to sweat blood. The medical term for this is hematohidrosis, which doctors believe is related to the body's fight-or-flight response. His emotional distress causes blood to trickle down his body. Still, he ultimately accepts what has to be done: "Yet not as I will, but as you will." Christ is able to accept whatever comes because he knows who his Father is. Like Heather, he's able to center his faith on who God is and what God has done.

And he knows that the God who created us out of his love will never abandon us, not even in death.

On a trip to Jerusalem after our first year of marriage, David and I visited this garden. We met a groundskeeper there who told me that the olive trees we were looking at were thousands of years old, meaning that they were the very trees Christ himself would've looked at while praying on that fateful night. As I stood in the garden, I felt a sense of peace wash over me. It was the end of a long day of sightseeing, of visiting various holy shrines that were thronged with other pilgrims. In the garden, though, David and I were some of the only people there, and I acutely felt the sense of God's loving, patient presence. When I got home, inspired by the garden's olive trees, I asked a friend to do a drawing of an olive branch. I went to a local tattoo shop and had the image engraved on my left forearm. When the tattoo artist finished, I held up my arm to the light and envisioned myself back in the garden. The tattoo reminds me that without lament, there isn't much reason for hope. It reminds me of Christ's humanity, that he is in my suffering with me.

* * *

David and I continued attending Resurrection services, and we made a point of attending all the post-service potlucks, where we got to know many of our fellow church members. I learned that several of the fifty or so members had come from backgrounds similar to David's and mine, which is to say they were looking for a new way to know and love God, free from the trauma of the past. There were students at Duke Divinity

School, and there were students at the medical school. There was a couple who had recently moved from Brooklyn. There was another couple who dyed fabrics and dreamed of owning their own farm. A theology student brought David and me to a local spot where he liked to go dancing. A biologist named Stephanie invited me to do a book study with her, and we started meeting regularly at a local coffee shop, where we discussed Soong-Chan Rah's *Prophetic Lament: A Call for Justice in Troubled Times.* From early on, I experienced Resurrection as a place where I could heal alongside others and feel safe for the first time in years.

Two months after we started attending Resurrection, I went to an Ash Wednesday service there. As a teenager, I never celebrated the holiday. There were parties and chocolate-shaped crosses, but never any reflections on what Jesus endured. I remember seeing a Catholic classmate with ashes smeared on his forehead and thinking that he needed to focus more on Christ's resurrection. No one had explained to me the meaning of the holiday and what we could learn from studying the sorrow of Jesus.

In the alleyway of a strip mall, members of my church glued a series of paper murals that depicted Jesus's path toward crucifixion. Two picnic tables sat in the alleyway, filled with people from my congregation writing in their notebooks or praying. The alleyway sat between a mental health clinic and a local grocery store. I had shown up late in my pajamas after forgetting to take my medications sprawled across the bathroom counter. Standing in the parking lot, Pastor Pat swept ash across my forehead and said: "For you are dust, and to dust you shall return."

To the people driving their cars hurriedly past this ceremony, this gesture may have seemed mundane, even archaic. For me, it was a tangible reminder of the fact that a life of faith could include suffering and sorrow. And there was a whole congregation around me, hearing these same words and grappling with the same questions that had followed me throughout my life. I felt a comfort I'd never felt before.

Over the course of that Ash Wednesday, I noticed people all over town with imperfectly drawn ash crosses on their foreheads, just like mine. People at the post office, people at the grocery store—I felt a kinship with them all. We were broken but still blessed. We were bound to die, but we lived with the promise of resurrection. I found comfort in these people with their ash-covered foreheads and their willingness to recognize all of this, without masking it with simple celebration.

* * *

One morning, about a year after I joined the Resurrection community, I attended a Bible study for women at the home of a fellow congregant named Sally, a retired schoolteacher from Florida. Before entering her home, I fidgeted in my car, flipping through my Bible like a student cramming before an important exam. I half expected Sally to test me on my knowledge and regretted the fact that I hadn't been more consistent in my reading of scripture. But I also knew why I'd taken time away from reading my Bible: I wanted a new start, free from old interpretations and painful associations.

Sally opened the door with a big smile and encouraged me to come on in. I walked into her living room and noticed several stacks of quilts and fabric scraps scattered across her couch. Photos of her grandchildren hung on the walls in every room. A group of older women about Sally's age sat around the dining room table with their Bibles and plates of pastries. I grabbed a scone and took an empty seat. Sally sat next to me and asked, "Would anyone like to say the opening prayer?" I stared at the floor, determined not to be called on. A woman wearing a sundress enthusiastically raised her hand and we bowed our heads as she spoke to God.

A few minutes into the Bible study, we heard a light tapping on the front door. Before Sally could answer, a woman named Lindy barged in. I heard the screen door slam, and then I saw Lindy drop her purse in the hall. She seemed to be lost in thought. She walked across the white carpet in her muddy sneakers, leaving a trail of footprints. I knew Lindy from church; sometimes, before services, she'd grab my blouse to study the stitching. She took the last seat at the table, touching every pastry on the platter before choosing the one remaining blueberry scone.

Sally tried to catch her up on what we were discussing, but Lindy swiftly interrupted her, talking about how she'd spent all day unpacking boxes of books for her new apartment down the road. She broke her scone into tiny pieces as crumbs fell across her lap. She acknowledged that she hadn't slept for days, and she then pulled out a piece of paper with a list of everything she'd organized in her new place. I felt a pang of recognition; I knew these symptoms well. We were witnessing a manic episode. I started to worry about how the other women would respond. Would they rush to try to fix her? Would they ask her to leave? I looked around the table, waiting for someone to quote a Bible verse about how God granted us peace, or for someone to grab Lindy by the shoulders and pray for her healing. That didn't happen. Instead, the other women sat quietly and listened. One woman offered to come by Lindy's new place the next day and help her continue unpacking. Lindy's face lit up, and she thanked her.

A church, at its best, is meant to carry God's presence into the world—to make the idea of God trustworthy. That was what these women were doing for Lindy, and for me, and for one another. Being part of this community didn't heal me, but it did point me toward a God who could be trusted, a God who met us in our frailty. Before we left Bible study, Sally passed around a prayer for us all to say together. I saw that it was Psalm 22, a prayer for help. Together, we read the words aloud: "But you, Lord, do not be far from me. You are my strength; come quickly to help me."

Chapter 11

One afternoon, while grabbing takeout from my favorite Thai restaurant, I got a phone call that I was too afraid to answer. Recently, at the urging of David and Dr. Paktar, I'd applied to some MFA programs. I didn't recognize the number, but I had a feeling it was from an admissions office, and I knew that the news was going to be bad. I pressed ignore and tried to think about my container of green curry. Then I saw that whoever had called had left a voicemail. I closed my eyes and pressed play.

It was the director of the Bennington Writing Seminars, a writing program in Vermont. "We've reviewed your application," he said, "and we'd love to see you join this upcoming January."

* * *

The Bennington Writing Seminars is a low-residency MFA program, which means students have to be physically on campus only two times per year, for ten days at a time. These ten-day stretches are called residencies, and they consist of lectures, writing workshops (when your fellow students give feedback on your work), and attempts at bonding with members of your call, also known as your cohort. The rest of the year, I would be responsible for writing twenty-five pages per month and corresponding with my professor.

When I arrived on campus for my first residency, I was struck by my good fortune. This was the fulfillment of a dream I'd had ever since Dr. Glidsan told me that I could write. And not only was *this* dream within reach, but so many others had come to pass. I was a married woman. I was a member of a church community that seemed reminiscent of home. I was a long way from the girl who thought that surviving into adulthood was the loftiest goal to which she could aspire.

Still, my normal pattern held. A good thing happened, and my mind started to persuade me that perhaps it was actually a bad thing. Or, worse yet, that it was a good thing I didn't deserve. I was on campus for less than a day when the bottom seemed to fall out again. Nothing on the outside had changed, but I'd learned long ago that the outside was seldom my problem. I frantically emailed Dr. Paktar. "I think I've made a terrible mistake," I wrote.

Pacing around my dorm room, I felt my phone vibrate; Dr. Paktar was calling. He encouraged me not to worry. He had a plan.

"I'm looking over your medication history," he said, "and I think we should consider ketamine treatment."

He told me that ketamine was a "dissociative anesthetic"— something that helps put you under for surgery—that was increasingly being tested for its antidepressant effects. It had not yet been approved by the FDA, and scientists weren't entirely sure how it worked. Some said it treated depression by reducing certain signals in the brain related to mood disorders, but the science was inconclusive. Still, Dr. Paktar assured me that the early results were promising, and he told me that he was opening a ketamine clinic in Charlotte, just two hours from where I lived. I agreed to the treatment for one simple reason: we were out of options. It's often when people have reached their lowest point that they become willing to take a leap of faith, and that was what it felt like I had to do. But first I had to get through my first residency.

*　*　*

Even though I was still taking medications as prescribed, I felt worse with each passing day. I stayed in my room as often as I could. Members of my cohort, people I'd just met, left notes under my door and brought me food. When I made it to lectures, I became too overwhelmed to sit through them. I stopped going to events on campus altogether.

During another phone call, Dr. Patkar explained that the medications I'd tried up until that point were designed to increase serotonin levels in my brain. My serotonin levels weren't the problem, though; my brain didn't have enough serotonin *receptors*, which rendered the drugs ineffective. One of his colleagues then gave me an evaluation over the phone that concluded what was already clear: I was depressed enough to receive ketamine treatment. I scheduled two weeks' worth of appointments at the ketamine center for when I returned home. My parents, well aware of my and David's financial situation, agreed to cover the costs of the treatment.

Before leaving my residency, I managed to make it to one meeting with my professor for that semester. I told him about the project I had in mind: an essay collection filled with extensive research about my family, including my great-grandmother Manoushag, who survived the Armenian genocide. He told me he was looking forward to working with me.

* * *

David and I arrived at the ketamine clinic after his GPS sent us to the end of a business park cul-de-sac, minutes away from Charlotte's bustling financial district. A receptionist greeted us as we entered, smiling and saying, "Right this way," before guiding us down a long hallway.

I'd brought my iPad with me so that I could watch *The Office* throughout the procedure. Inside the treatment room there were two suede recliner chairs, the kind you might use to watch a football game, and David and I sat in them. I pulled the lever back to recline, and a group of doctors walked in, one pushing an IV cart that held a plastic bag filled with ketamine. In his free hand he held a binder, which I noticed had the number "1" written on the spiral, indicating that I was the clinic's first patient. I later learned that Dr. Patkar had been so worried about me that he got me in before the clinic officially opened.

"On a scale of one to ten," one of the doctors asked, "what is your desire to die?"

I glanced quickly at David and gave an honest answer: "Nine."

The doctor adjusted his glasses and said, "There's hope for the future."

I laughed, feeling the absurdity of my situation. I felt that I had experienced enough of the highs and lows of my illness to know that the future wouldn't be bright. The memories of the good times only made the pain of relapse more acute. Those times when medication *worked*, now lost to the past, made the thought of going on this way unbearable. Despite the doctor's words, at that moment I felt like a deeply hopeless case.

A nurse wearing a blue pair of latex gloves walked into the room and rubbed my arm with alcohol. I looked away to keep from seeing the size of the needle that she was carrying. As she inserted the needle, I pictured iron nails being hammered into Christ's hands as his body was fastened onto a wooden cross—a favorite coping mechanism of mine. Imagining the sound of the nails crushing through bone and muscle kept me from wincing. Once the needle was securely in my vein, the nurse dimmed the lights and left the room.

The procedure lasted an hour, but I can't recall much of it. I felt high within ten to fifteen minutes. Episodes of *The Office* seemed especially vivid, and I kept pausing and rewinding to point out details that had eluded me in the first hundred or so times I'd watched the show. David recorded a video of me laughing uncontrollably and saying, "Do you think I'm *The Office*'s target audience?" This seemed an important question at the time. I looked around the room, searching for the doctor. My eyes filled with happy tears, and I said, "You cured me!"

I returned to the clinic two more times that week. After the third session, when the doctor asked me to rate my desire to die on a scale of one to ten, I said, "Two." This wasn't an attempt to downplay my symptoms; this was the truth. My thoughts of death were gone.

On the ride home, sitting in the passenger seat as David drove, I tried to recall my repetitive, intrusive thoughts about death, but I couldn't. Instead, it was though the world outside my head, the world I actually lived in, was forcing its way into my consciousness. I noticed the trees along the highway with their brightly colored leaves, indicating the changing of the seasons. I noticed the clouds overhead. I read every billboard we passed, every street sign. I scanned the rear bumpers of cars for funny bumper stickers—no luck, but I kept looking. For the first time in months, I was able to see the world again, to take in all the little details. I wished I had a pad and pencil with me so I could start writing a poem.

In the weeks that followed, I started wearing bright colors and reaching out to friends again. When I was with friends, I found that I could actually be with them. I could listen to them. I could ask about their lives.

My mom calling my recovery a miracle inspired me to re-visit the Gospel accounts of the miracles of Jesus. When Jesus heals people of physical symptoms, he does not alleviate their painful memories. The blind man Jesus cures in the Gospel of John had been blind for his entire life; in his new life of sight, he will still carry with him the experience of his blindness. The story of Jesus healing the paraplegic man is recounted in all four Gospels, and they all agree that Jesus grants the man the ability to walk. But they don't tell us about his long walk home, a walk that I'm sure included reflection on the decades when he could not move unassisted. Even Jesus himself after his resurrection is still marked by the wounds of crucifixion. Ketamine had indeed relieved my symptoms in a way that felt

miraculous—but I still grieved the time lost, and I still con-
templated the darkness I survived.

* * *

A few months later, I had a follow-up appointment in which
I received a fresh infusion of ketamine and met with a psychiatrist tasked with evaluating my progress. Looking over my
charts and questionnaires, he concluded that I didn't need my
extensive medication regimen anymore. "Ketamine," he said,
"is enough to control your moods."

When I told Dr. Patkar about the doctor's assessment during
our next appointment, he disagreed immediately. "Anna," he
said, "you're always going to need to be on medication to
manage your symptoms."

Even so, I flushed some pills down the toilet and began
tapering from others. It's hard for me to assess what went
through my mind exactly when making such a drastic decision.
Individuals understandably do not want to live with side effects like gaining dozens of pounds, difficulty having orgasms,
or being endlessly tired at all hours. But I wanted to believe
that ketamine had cured me. On some level, I suspect I also
wanted to be free of the daily reminders of my bipolar disorder, which the act of taking my pills each morning represented.

* * *

After six months of ketamine treatment, I traveled to Vermont in June 2018 for my second residency without packing
any medications, determined to be free of them. I struggled
from the beginning to make any of the lectures or workshops.

During one writing workshop, we were dissecting an essay about a swarm of locusts invading the Horn of Africa, and my thoughts, without warning, returned to the prospect of my death. As the discussion continued—"Add a scene here," one student said; "I really like this narrator," another said—I was besieged by the desire to end my own life. The thoughts played over and over again: End it. End it. I grabbed my purse and went out the door, without any explanation. I noticed my whole body was dripping sweat. I went down some stairs, looking for someone who could help me. An administrator from the program led me into an office and told me there was a nearby hospital she could take me to. I shook my head and told her I had to call my psychiatrist. I stepped into the hall and called Dr. Patkar.

"I haven't been taking my medications correctly," I told him. "I thought the ketamine had cured me."

He sighed. "Please send me the information for your local pharmacy," he said. "I'm going to call in your prescriptions." The pharmacy would have them by morning; now I had to get through the rest of the day.

That night, while writing in my room, the suicidal thoughts worsened. I decided that I was going to get a ride to the hospital—an absolute last resort, because Dr. Paktar had always worried that a hospital stay would be traumatic for me and possibly result in my getting overmedicated. As I walked to my door, I heard a friend, a member of my cohort named Davin, call my name from across the hall.

"Do you want to go for a walk around campus with me?" he said. "It seems like you've had a long day."

I followed him without thinking and without mentioning my intention to check myself into the hospital. As we walked, he started telling me about a short story he'd been working on, and I asked him questions about the characters. We sat in the quad in silence, and he scratched the side of his beard, the way he still does when he's thinking. In the distance we saw some students sitting around a bonfire, and we could hear them talking and laughing. The fire's flames shed just enough light that I could see the faint outlines of mountains on the horizon. A swarm of fireflies appeared over our heads like a rain cloud. We sat for minutes without speaking, staring up at the sky.

There have been so many moments throughout my life when people's kindness, people's simple presence, has saved me. This was another such moment, and it was a reminder of God's presence in my difficult moments. It's hard to see Davin's invitation to go for a walk as anything other than a miracle. Lying in my bed that night, I pictured the flickering light.

The next morning, an administrator from the college drove me to the pharmacy to pick up my prescriptions. Two other friends, James and Billy, took me for lunch at a local diner. The medications started to kick in, and I was feeling more like myself.

It was around this time that the direction of my writing started to shift. My professor had been supportive of my initial project—the family history—but he suspected that this wasn't my real topic, at least not now. He encouraged me to go deep into my experience of faith and mental illness, to really look at it, to see what light I could find.

To graduate from Bennington, I had to complete a lecture on a topic of my choice, do a reading of my original work, and submit a thesis. I returned to Vermont in January 2020 to do just that.

Before my reading, I stood at the podium and looked out across the lecture hall. I saw so many people there who'd carried me, whose support had sustained me—friends who'd responded to my anxious texts, friends who'd stayed up late to watch films about faith with me, professors who'd helped me go deeper into my faith and my work. These people, too, were my church. Thanks to them, my losses had not brought me disaster. I read an essay about my diagnosis, but in the back of my mind, I was offering a prayer of thanks: *Lord, you delivered me.*

The graduation ceremony was held on a dark, cold evening, snow covering every inch of campus. David flew up to be there, and my parents made the trip from Michigan where they had recently relocated to be near their parents. The commencement speaker was Jericho Brown, a poet I had read and admired while I was at Hope. The part of his speech that struck me was about a tree he had loved as a child, a tree whose details had stayed with him. I thought again of the guidance I'd received from Dr. Glidsan, the first teacher who told me I was a writer: Focus on those details. Bring out those details. Write what only you can write. Later that night, as I held my diploma, I remembered the letter I'd written to myself during my first week at Hope, which I'd recently gotten in the mail.

"Dear Anna," it read, "I think that you might be okay."

Chapter 12

One night that fall, well into a pandemic that had upended life around the world, I lifted the glass lid on a pan on our stove and immediately thought I was going to throw up. David saw my face and asked what the matter was. "It's just grilled pork," he said. I walked over and opened our kitchen windows, trying to rid myself of the smell. "Shut them," David said. "You're letting bugs in."

"I feel like I'm going to get sick," I replied.

He walked over to the cabinet and handed me a cup of Pepto-Bismol. I plugged my nose and chugged the pink liquid.

In the weeks that followed, I woke up every morning physically exhausted and nauseated, and I remained nauseated until after lunch. I normally went to the gym every morning, but each session left me out of breath and needing to take a nap. Foods that I ate daily like chicken or berry smoothies suddenly seemed disgusting, and I replaced them with saltines and sesame bagels. This went on for weeks. One morning, while David and I were out walking our pit bull mutt, I complained again about my fatigue. "Maybe I need to go get a Covid test," I said.

"It's more likely that you're pregnant," David replied.

We laughed. We both assumed for years that I didn't have

the ability to have children. Since my diagnosis, my menstrual cycle was never consistent, and I'd go months and even years without having a period. Pregnancy seemed to be out of the question. We were early in the process of pursuing adoption. A few days later, I woke up early to go to the gym and felt heavy cramping. David was out for a run, and I decided I'd go to the pharmacy to get a pregnancy test, just to rule out the possibility. I didn't trust myself to be able to accurately read a plus or minus sign, so I bought a digital test, one that would simply read: PREGNANT.

When I got home, David was back from his run and had gone upstairs to his office to work. I went straight to the bathroom. Minutes later, as I stared down at the test, the answer was clear: I was pregnant. I stared at the test for minutes, making sure the word wasn't going to disappear. I wondered if maybe the test was faulty, so I took the other one in the box. There it was again: PREGNANT. For a fleeting moment, I thought about coming up with a cute way to tell David I was pregnant, searching my mind for the many examples of pregnancy-reveal videos I'd seen on YouTube. But that thought gave way to a simple imperative, which was that I needed David to calm me down. I ran upstairs and found David at his desk, staring at his computer screen.

"David," I said.

He turned around, and I stuck the pregnancy tests in his face. "Oh wow," he said. He wrapped his arms around my waist. I latched on to him, unwilling to let go. He looked down at my face and wiped tears from my eyes.

"What do we do now?" he said.

"I need to hear the baby's heartbeat to know this is happening."

I looked up nearby women's health centers on my phone and, insisting that I go alone, I got in the car to drive to the nearest one.

* * *

I didn't realize until arriving at the center that it was a Christian pregnancy center, the type I've always associated with the pro-life movement. In my mind, Christian pregnancy centers are designed to give moms with unwanted pregnancies the resources to prevent abortions while subtly delivering the news of Jesus. As I walked in the door, I expected that the people working there would see my panic and rush to talk me out of an abortion. An older woman ran toward the door and smiled at me.

"What brings you in here today?" she said.

"I took a pregnancy test at home, and I want an ultrasound to see the baby."

"So does that mean that you're keeping the baby?"

"Yes, of course I am."

I could see the relief on her face when I said this. She led me down a hallway with walls covered in Bible verses detailing the sanctity of life and took me into an office and shut the door. The woman ran her fingers through bangs coated in hairspray and sat down across from me. She asked about my symptoms. After I finished listing off what I had described to David for six weeks, she admitted they did not have an ultrasound machine but offered to give me another pregnancy test. I took a deep breath and leaned my head back on the couch.

All I wanted was to hear my baby's heartbeat. It turned out that the center existed only to confirm pregnancies for women and offer adoption services, counseling, and support programs for families. Medical treatment was not available. I shrugged and said, "Sure, why not."

I received my third positive test result of the day. "Congratulations!" the woman said, hugging me as I stood stiff with my arms at my sides. She packed me a bag of prenatal vitamins and handed me a pamphlet about Jesus Christ before sending me on my way.

* * *

Abraham is considered the patriarch of what are known as the Abrahamic religions: Judaism, Christianity, and Islam. For Christians, he is a prophet, a man with a special relationship with God. Saint Augustine wrote that Christians are all children of Abraham.

Abraham's story is recounted in the book of Genesis. He has a wife, Sarah, who is unable to have children. When she turns ninety, God speaks to Abraham and tells him, "I will bless her and will surely give you a son by her." In response, Abraham falls on the ground laughing. This was unfathomable to him. When Sarah learns the news, she also laughs. But the truth was the truth: Sarah was indeed pregnant. They name their child Isaac, Hebrew for "one who laughs."

Had God told me during any of my depressive episodes that I was to become a mother, I also would have laughed.

* * *

I was never sure I wanted to be a mom, mainly because I was so afraid that my mental health would have a negative impact on my children. I would never want my child, someone utterly reliant on me, to see me unable to get out of bed or manically rearranging the furniture in the house. I'd read my share of memoirs about bad mothers; in darker moments, I imagined the memoir my future child would write about me.

Driving home from the pregnancy center, the reality of my situation started to sink in. David and I were going to have a child. In doing so, we were choosing to side with hope. That's what it is to bring a new life into this world: a radical statement of hope. Or at least that was how I felt that day, driving by the familiar sights of my neighborhood that now shone with new vividness, because they would be the sights that my child would see, sights I hoped my child would come to love. My tendency to dwell on global doom was momentarily set aside. This was a messy world, yes, and it can be filled with such sorrow. But my faith had taught me to see—and to know—that a light shone even in the darkness.

As soon as I got home from the pregnancy center, I prepared to FaceTime Dr. Patkar. As soon as his face appeared on my phone screen, I shouted, "I'm pregnant!"

His jaw dropped, and then he said, "That's great news! You're going to be a great mother."

I burst into tears. He told me that he needed to adjust my medications but that I would be fine. I couldn't stop crying. I asked him if the hormones would send me into a manic episode, and he shook his head and told me stories about other patients who had enjoyed perfectly stable and healthy pregnancies.

Two weeks later, David and I went to an initial obstetrician appointment. As the technician rubbed the transducer across my stomach, we both looked at the screen and listened. There it was: a heartbeat. David gasped and held my hand. Our black Covid masks prevented me from seeing David's reaction, but I could see the wrinkles around his eyes that he gets when he smiles. Both of our families lived hundreds of miles away, so we didn't have anyone nearby to celebrate with us. But we still felt that we had everything we needed.

Two months into my pregnancy, I received a writing residency in a cabin at a farm fifteen minutes away from our house. In the afternoons, I left home and spent several hours writing about the faith of my childhood. The farm owners had two children who played outside in the woods. One afternoon, I walked through those woods, filled with paths that the family created for others to hike around their yard. The owners' daughter, who was around five and kept her hair in uneven pigtails, led me to a fort made of sticks that she foraged for days and climbed inside. The kids ran around, using their imaginations to pretend that they had their own village deep in the forest. I watched the young girl dance and thought of my own child running through the woods with me. As I stood there, a Bible verse came to mind: "The Lord is my rock, and my fortress, and my deliverer" (Psalms 18:2). I placed my hand on my stomach and imagined feeling my child kick for the first time.

A few weeks later, my sister paid for me to go get another

ultrasound. A nurse led David and me into a dark room and had me lie across the table. She brought in the ultrasound machine and set up a large screen where we saw images of our child.

"You're having a girl!" she said.

David looked at me. "Anna, how do you feel?"

"Scared."

* * *

Every week, I met with a therapist named Elizabeth to discuss my fears of motherhood. During one session, I told her about my fears in regards to raising my daughter in the church, my fears that my daughter would be traumatized in the way I was.

"All your daughter needs to know," she said, "is that God loves her."

Over the course of my pregnancy, I developed a renewed interest in theology. I wanted to understand God in a new way. Elizabeth pointed out to me that faith, for many people, is a meaningful hedge against fear. But my faith—my belief in God—has long been a major source of fear in my life. She used the term *religious trauma* to describe the impact that faith had historically had on me. One night, while David played video games, I told him about some of the theology I'd been reading, explaining that many early Christians didn't believe in hell as it's commonly understood, but rather saw it as a metaphor for our suffering here on earth. When David asked if that meant I no longer believed in hell, I said, "I don't know what I believe about hell, or about a lot of things. I'm learning to be okay with that."

I turned back to my book I was reading. It was about Isaac of Nineveh, also known as Isaac the Syrian. He was a seventh-century bishop in the Eastern church and a theologian who found the notion of eternal hell to be incompatible with a loving God. He believed that all of creation would be saved. This thought comforted me. I felt even more comforted by the fact that Christians, dating back centuries, have struggled with these big questions.

Reading about the life of Isaac didn't give me greater confidence in my parenting abilities. But it did give me confidence in the reality of God's love. That was the framework I wanted to share with my daughter. And my prayer for her was that she wouldn't have to spend years of her life striving to earn the Lord's favor. My prayer was that she could rest in the reality that she was already enough.

A Letter to Ezra

Every day after I found out I was pregnant, your father and I would walk around the neighborhood after lunch and talk about what we wanted to name you. We watched neighbors drive by as we discussed the eccentric new names that Hollywood stars were giving their kids, names like Apple, North, Maple, Sunday. Your father and I have different tastes when it comes to most things, so it's no surprise that we didn't come to a swift conclusion. Your father assumed that I wanted to give you a name from a novel or a poem, or maybe the name of a powerful woman from history. Your father ended up being the one to choose your name.

"What about Ezra?" he said one morning, as our dog led us onto someone's manicured front lawn. I immediately said, "Okay," which caught your father by surprise. As we continued to walk, he grabbed my hand.

I researched your name when I got home. I learned Ezra was a Hebrew word for "helper." Thinking about how God had helped and protected your father and me throughout our marriage, the name struck me as perfect.

Then there's the book of Ezra. Part of the Old Testament, it tells a story of restoration. The Jewish people see their kingdom destroyed, but they believe that their God is faithful.

After years of exile, a prophet named Ezra leaves Babylon to rebuild Jerusalem. To restore their kingdom and to build a new temple that will bear witness to God's goodness. The story of Ezra is a story of destruction and rebuilding, of death and resurrection. It's a story that makes sense of so much of my and your father's lives, and our lives together.

When your father and I told our couples therapist about your name, she placed her hand over her chest. "The name says so much about the restoration you continue to seek," she said.

The restoration your father and I seek—that we continue to seek, even now—is to an idea of God that we want to teach to you, one free from the beliefs we want to protect you from. In that way, through this restoration, we can be the parents you deserve.

Because the pandemic prevented us from traveling, your father and I spent Christmas at home for the first time since getting married. We couldn't help but wonder what the next Christmas would be like with you here. I imagined your hands on the ornaments on the tree, looking at the lights with awe. Your father and I walked through the woods for miles, my jacket barely fitting over my belly. The trail was empty, since everyone else was busy at home with their families. We spent Christmas night rolling Armenian dumplings made from a recipe given to me by your great-grandmother Manoushag. I finished the dumplings, bringing the ceramic bowl up to my mouth and tipping my head back so I could drink every last drop of broth. All throughout the meal, I felt you kick.

The headlines were filled with troubling news—more Covid deaths, no end to the pandemic in sight, racial and political divides, church scandals. Sometimes we felt hopeless, but you helped us. You carried us through. I would hold my stomach and think of Jesus's mother, Mary, forced to give birth in a manger. Maybe she had the same anxieties I had about bringing a new life into the world. But now I know for sure what Mary felt when she first held her baby in her arms—a love that overflowed.

Whenever I worried about you and the world you would be born into, I thought about everything I wanted to share with you. I wanted you to one day feel the breeze as we hold hands and walk down the beach at night, watching the sky turn black and fill with stars. I wanted you to one day see the flowers at my favorite garden, blossoming as the spring season dawns. I wanted the beauty of this world to overtake you, to sustain you, to help you get through another day. I wanted you to see everything that can convince you that life is so much more than pain, that the real meaning of our lives is found in the gracious beauty that surrounds us.

But I still had to bring you into the world. One week before you were born, I went to my appointment and the doctor placed a fetal doppler over my stomach to measure your heartbeat.

"You must be pretty miserable, huh," he said.

My ankles were barely visible from the swelling; I felt my thighs sticking together wherever I walked. I could never find a position at night that was comfortable enough to keep me asleep. I told the doctor that I was ready to give birth, that it was time.

"The best I can do," he said, "is to induce you one day before your due date."

I counted this as a victory. Your dad and I made plans to eat at all our favorite restaurants one last time before you arrived. We followed every craving: tacos, cookies covered in frosting, cheeseburgers, gyros, pasta smothered in alfredo. But things didn't go as planned. Three days before my scheduled induction, I felt stomach cramps. Your dad assured me that it was nothing. By the time he fell asleep, I realized that this felt different. Timing my contractions on my phone, I realized I was going into labor.

The birthing classes I took to prepare for your arrival taught me all these different movements and exercises to do in labor, but I didn't want to do any of that. All I wanted was to lay on the giant beanbag that your dad bought me and eat a piece of toast smothered with salted butter. I didn't want to wake up your dad in case I was wrong, so I waited just until my phone app told me to get ready for the hospital. I walked into our bedroom, leaned over his side of the bed, and tapped him on the shoulder.

"I'm in labor," I said. "I need you to wake up."

He kept his eyes closed and put the covers over his head. "Okay," he said. "Will you go make us some coffee?"

I can tell you this: For as long as he lives, your father will not live that one down. One thing to know about him is how heavily he relies on his daily routine. He told me that since we would be in the hospital all day, he was going to go for a short run. "I promise I'll be back in time," he said. I kept looking at my watch, but somehow he made it home right as my contractions were coming closer together.

As we entered the hospital, a nurse brought over a wheelchair even though I insisted that I could walk. David took my shoulders and led me to a wheelchair. "You need to rest," he said. I looked up in disdain, wanting to prove my strength. They took us to a room for me to be evaluated, which was when I began screaming in pain. My body leaned sideways in the bed as my hands clung to its metal sides. I closed my eyes, trying to focus on my breathing. My entire body became drenched in sweat.

"I need you to go get an epidural as fast as you can," I said.

But it was not that simple. They placed me in a pair of stirrups and announced, "You're five centimeters dilated. You came here just in time." Your dad made a joke about how this was the first instance in my life that I was not at least ten minutes late. I asked for your estimated time of arrival, and the nurse told us you might be here by noon. Five hours from when we arrived.

Once we had our own room, an anesthesiologist walked in to give me my requested epidural. Within moments, the painful contractions disappeared. I pulled out my phone and ordered some clothes for you. At 6:00 p.m., well past noon, I ordered myself a turkey sandwich from the deli nearby.

The nurses instructed me to get in various positions on the bed to help my cervix open more. Your dad kept looking away because he knew how much pain I was in as I repositioned myself; it felt like I was in some sort of torturous yoga class. The doctor walked in, grabbed a sharp object, and stuck it up inside of me. As soon as she did, I grabbed the sides of the bed and screamed in pain.

"Okay, you should be ready to push soon," she said.

Preparing myself for what was about to happen, I took a deep breath. Your dad stood next to me and grabbed my hand. He told me to pretend that I was preparing to complete a workout, and I pictured myself doing burpees at the gym and the sandwich I'd soon eat. I was relearning a lesson life had shown me over and over again, a lesson you will learn, too: pain can exist alongside joy. Because, Ezra, joy is exactly what I felt, knowing you'd soon be with us. Scripture often describes creation itself as a woman laboring in anticipation of the new world to come, the new life to come. I pushed and pushed again, and there you were: Ezra Jane Gazmarian. You were born on July 7, 2021, eight years to the day after I put a garden gnome on your father's front porch in an attempt to get him to date me. The doctors placed you in my arms and kept talking, and your father placed his hands on us both, but I was focused only on you. The features I'd never seen on another human face, already uniquely yours. My daughter. While we both lay there, your dad fed me the best turkey sandwich ever made. We lay there for over an hour. This was a holy time.

And the time since then, now that you've just turned two—that, too, has been holy time. Your existence is a gift to me and to your father. A daily reminder of God's goodness. There have been times in the past two years when my mental health has taken one of those turns I've come to expect, times when I can barely function—and there you are, stomping around the living room, playing with your stuffed dog, and saying, "It's okay, Mommy." I see the way you take in the world, absorbing all the little details, and I remember that these are the moments that are most important to God.

It's true, Ezra, that we live in a world that gives us plenty of reasons to be fearful and doubtful. I wish I could shield you from every last hardship, to take on any pain you'll ever feel as my own. The best I can do is to remind you of what I've come to know—that this world also gives us plenty of reasons to stop, pay attention, and let awe overwhelm us. That you will meet people over the course of your journey—teachers, friends, pastors, workout partners—who will help you remember who you are, and be the presence of God for you, just as so many have done for me. Beyond that, there's not much I can say for sure. I don't know.

What I do know is that tonight you climbed in bed between your father and me, and you demanded that your father read a bedtime story. You prefer his reading voice to mine, and I can't blame you. As he read, you pointed to every page, mumbling words that I couldn't quite understand, at least not yet. And tomorrow, God willing, your father and I will lie out on the front lawn and watch as you run in circles, laughing with joyful abandon, full of trust.

Resources

Books

Kaveh Akbar (editor), *The Penguin Book of Spiritual Verse: 110 Poets on the Divine*

Beth Allison Barr, *The Making of Biblical Womanhood*

Rachel Held Evans, *Inspired: Slaying Giants, Walking on Water, and Loving the Bible Again*

Rachel Held Evans, *Searching for Sunday: Loving, Leaving, and Finding the Church*

Katie Ford, *If You Have to Go: Poems*

David Bentley Hart, *That All Shall Be Saved*

Kay Redfield Jamison, *An Unquiet Mind: A Memoir of Moods and Madness*

Leslie Jamison, *The Empathy Exams*

Hillary L. McBride, *The Wisdom of Your Body*

Kristin Kobes du Mez, *Jesus and John Wayne: How White Evangelicals Corrupted a Faith and Fractured a Nation*

Yiyun Li, *Dear Friend, from My Life I Write to You in Your Life*

Brennan Manning, *The Ragamuffin Gospel: Good News for the Bedraggled, Beat-Up, and Burnt Out*

Thomas Merton, *The Wisdom of the Desert*

Soong-Chan Rah, *Prophetic Lament: A Call for Justice in Troubled Times*

Esmé Weijun Wang, *The Collected Schizophrenias*

Rowan Williams, *Tokens of Trust: An Introduction to Christian Belief*

Christian Wiman, *My Bright Abyss: Meditation of a Modern Believer*

Lauren F. Winner, *Still: Notes on a Mid-Faith Crisis*

Nicholas Wolterstorff, *Lament for a Son*

Podcasts
The Deconstructionists
Exvangelical
Good Faith
The Hilarious World of Depression
Holy/Hurt Podcast
Holy Post
The Liturgists
Nomad
The Rise and Fall of Mars Hill
Straight White American Jesus
Terrible, Thanks For Asking
Voxology

Research

Bahji, Anees, Carlos A. Zarate, and Gustavo H. Vazquez. "Ketamine for Bipolar Depression: A Systematic Review." *International Journal of Neuropsychopharmacology* 24, no. 7 (July 2021): 535–41.

Gitlin, M. J., et al. "Relapse and Impairment in Bipolar Disorder." *The American Journal of Psychiatry* 152, no. 11 (November 1995): 1635–40.

Kessler, Ronald C., et al. "Age of Onset of Mental Disorders: A Review of Recent Literature." *Current Opinion in Psychiatry* 20, no. 4 (July 2007): 359–64.

Laursen, Thomas Munk. "Life Expectancy Among Persons with Schizophrenia or Bipolar Affective Disorder." *Schizophrenia Research* 131, no. 1–3 (September 2011): 101–04.

Little, Alison. "Treatment-Resistant Depression." *American Family Physician* 80, no. 2 (July 2009): 167–72.

Rihmer, Zoltán, Xénia Gonda, and Péter Döme. "The Assessment and Management of Suicide Risk in Bipolar Disorder." In André F. Carvalho and Eduard Vieta, editors. *The Treatment of Bipolar Disorder: Integrative Clinical Strategies and Future Directions*. Oxford: Oxford University Press, 2017.

Salvi, Virginio, et al. "ADHD and Bipolar Disorder in Adulthood: Clinical and Treatment Implications." *Medicina (Kaunas, Lithuania)* 57, no. 5 (May 2021): 466.

Shin, Cheolmin, and Yong-Ku Kim. "Ketamine in Major Depressive Disorder: Mechanisms and Future Perspectives." *Psychiatry Investigation* 17, no. 3 (March 2020): 181–92.

Souery, Daniel, George I. Papakostas, and Madhukar H. Trivedi. "Treatment-Resistant Depression." *Journal of Clinical Psychiatry* 67, supplement 6 (2006): 16–22.

Torrent, Carla, et al. "Cognitive Impairment in Bipolar II Disorder." *The British Journal of Psychiatry* 189, no. 3 (September 2006): 254–59.

Acknowledgments

I used to think of writing as an isolating and solitary act. But as I wrote this book, I learned the vital nature of community for my work. This book would not be possible without the people in my life who inspired many of these pages with their experiences and stories. I see the clearest depiction of God through those who have loved and supported me during this process.

Yahdon Israel, you took a complete leap of faith in wanting my book even before I had an agent. I'll never forget falling over in my bathroom at nine months pregnant when speaking on the phone with you for the first time, realizing that my dreams were coming true. Thank you for seeing the nuances and complexities of faith that I wanted to explore. You saw the potential of this book before I could. I am grateful for the time and patience you put into developing these pages, especially on days when I was running on about three hours of sleep with a newborn.

To every individual at Simon & Schuster who helped with this book, from exchanging emails about production to designing a book cover that made me pull over on the side of the road when I saw it for the first time because of how perfect it is, thank you for your help in making the book of my dreams.

Billy Glidden, I don't even know where to begin. Thank you for the creative partnership and friendship that has challenged me and made me a better writer. I already miss our late-night phone calls when we yelled about minor details that most readers won't notice. Your peace balances out my chaos. Every edit you made was tied to my vision for this book, and that's the greatest gift that I could ask for.

Andrea Walker, you were the first editor to work with me on this project and helped me develop a road map for several of my future books and what I hope to accomplish as a writer.

Cassie Mannes Murray, I knew that I wanted to work with you from the moment we had pancakes for the first time. Thank you for selling this book and for your friendship.

Danielle Bukowski, thank you for walking through this editorial process with me, being an incredible advocate, and, most importantly, teaching me to dream big. I could not ask for a more supportive agent.

Susanna Childress, I have learned so much from you as a teacher, mentor, and close friend. You were one of the first people to believe in my writing, and this book never would have happened without your support and trail mix bags in class. Most of all, you have taught me the important truth that excelling as a writer is not enough; you must also excel at kindness. Thank you for modeling this for me and everyone in your life.

Jane Gerbrandt, when we were sixteen and I didn't know how to fill up the gas in my new car, I called you, and you immediately drove to the gas station. That's exactly the type of friend you need to walk through life with, especially while writing a book. Thanks for reading every poetry draft and my early work, for being my first editor. Thank you for staying, for praying, for driving with me for hours with Bon Iver playing, even though I am a terrible driver. Your presence and prayers are why I am still here. Here's to another sixteen years of friendship.

Bethie Figgie, thank you for teaching me about the importance of being present in times of need, for walking through Target with me late at night, loving my child, sending me pug photos, driving long distances for good pastries, sitting in strip mall parking lots with me, and cheering me on every step of the way of this process. You have taught me so much about friendship.

Davin Malasarn, you will always be my MFA husband. Thank you for the many baked goods to encourage and celebrate me. I appreciate your patience in putting up with my editorial procrastination tendencies in sending you dozens of photos of dresses and food. Your loyalty over the years has kept me believing that one day this whole book thing could happen. Guess what? Yours comes out next.

Margo Steines, I feel like I've known you for thirty years. Thank you for going through the book process before me and for your guidance. You are the only person who will talk to me about protein powder, writing, bamboo toddler clothing, and dumbbells. Grateful.

Molly House, I survived early motherhood while writing a book because of you. Thank you for answering every one of my questions about sleep regressions, swaddling, and baby development. You were basically my daughter's personal WebMD. Also, texts about reality television were appreciated.

ACKNOWLEDGMENTS

Thanks to my teachers who have patiently endured my tangential emails and run-on sentences. You helped me find my voice and fall in love with literature, two things that I can never repay you for: Heather Sellers, Pablo Peschiera, Peter Trachtenberg, Clifford Thompson, Craig Teicher Morgan, Dinah Lenney, Stephen Hemenway, and Kendra Parker.

Chris and Rachel Breslin, Meg Hoffman, Gwen Heginbotham, Rachel Rivers, Stephanie Holmer, Elizabeth Christensen, and my church community: Thank you for creating a space of safety and healing for me to wrestle with God. Thank you for helping me have hope in what the church can be.

For Burn North Durham, thank you for giving me a space to show up and get stronger physically, emotionally, mentally, and spiritually. Thanks to my trainers Sarah Amodeo, Jo Nocito, and Cheryl Dickerson for pushing me beyond what I ever think is possible. For my workout buddies who secretly love burpees as much as I do and have supported me in every way: Kim Arrington, Laurie Hyland, Amber Stohl, and every other woman at my gym.

For my writer friends who kept me writing: Molly Guinn Bradley, Millie Ferguson, Ryan Matthews, James McGinniss, Lisa Cockrel, John West, Nicole Treska, Robert James Russell, Kevin Koczwara, Garrett Bucks, Barbara Sostaita, Natalie Lima, Nick Lawson, Kyle Smith, Suleika Jaouad, Doug Jones, Camille Dungy, Leslie Jamison, Rachel Yoder, Emily Maloney, Cameron Dezen Hammon, Pat Megley, Frank Pagliaro, Hillary L. McBride, Kyle Smith, Emily Rapp Black, Allyson Hoffman, and my amazing apocalyptic cohort.

To my favorite poetry classmates: Michael Reynolds, Laura

Kraay, Connor Hughes, Eric Dawson, Alex Mouw, Anne Hasa, April Johnson, Taylor Rebhan, and everyone else who endured many of my shitty poems about purity rings.

To the childcare workers and neighbors who watched my daughter from when she was three months old, which enabled me to write this book: the Knelsons, Stacey Wallen, Ayla Smart, Lauren Seale, Kristi Meter, Jenna Settlage, Suzi Brynes, Nurtured Baby, and Our Playhouse. This book would not be possible without your loving care.

Thanks to my coworkers at *The Sun* magazine for being extremely gracious with me during book deadlines. Working with you makes me a better writer.

To my Glam Squad for prioritizing my mental health: Dr. Ashwin Patkar, Avance Psychiatry, Whitney Johnson, Elizabeth Harrison, Mackenzie Almond, Charlotte Donlon, Jenna Horgan, Carlye Schroeder, my wonderful group at Welwynn, and my family at Sierra Tuscon. Thank you for listening.

Thank you to Bennington Writing Seminars, Queens Book Development Program, and Down Yonder Farm for giving me the time to write.

To my favorite places to write while my infant napped: Cocoa Cinnamon, Joe Van Gogh, and Namu—you gave me the caffeine and inspiration that I needed.

To the musical artists who served as the soundtrack of this book: Sufjan Stevens, Julien Baker, Lucy Dacus, and the National.

Mom and Dad, I doubt that any parent is especially thrilled to hear that their kid is getting a degree in creative writing without any clear career path or that they aspire to write a memoir dealing with their childhood. But throughout this process, you have supported me in numerous ways and believed fully that I was following my calling. Thank you for helping me get the healthcare that I needed and enabling me to get necessary treatment. I would not be where I am in life without you.

Allie Miller, your support, honesty, and kindness in guiding me through motherhood has sustained me. Thank you for being my sister.

Ezra Gazmarian, I started revising this book on the day that I got home from the hospital with you. I learned the art of holding a newborn while typing with one hand. Your life and the life of this book are deeply connected. Thank you for who you are and the joy that you bring to everyone you meet. Whenever I stepped away from my computer after a long day of editing, finding you putting your dogs down for a nap, singing songs, or dancing brought me back to living in the present—and what a gift.

David Gazmarian, my love, none of this would be possible without you. I told you on our first date that I was going to write a book, and you made sacrifices throughout our time together to make this happen. Thank you for the life that you have built with me, for your partnership, for being an amazing father, for making meals, for listening to me read draft upon draft for years before we knew I'd ever get a book deal. You always had faith that my dreams would come true. This book deals with painful times in our marriage, and revisiting those periods was hard on us both. Your perseverance, patience, and humor sustained me throughout the process. The pies, cakes, cookies, and pastries that you made me also helped. I love you.

Anna Gazmarian holds an MFA in creative writing from the Bennington Writing Seminars. Her essays have been published in *The Sun* magazine, *The Guardian*, *The Rumpus*, and *Longreads*. She works for *The Sun* and lives with her family in Durham, North Carolina.